BLESSED

My Battle with Brain Disease

Mary J. Stevens

Mary J. Stevens

To the praise and glory of God, Who has continuously showered blessings upon me and Who has guided and directed me throughout my life and in writing this book.

Also, to my hero, my husband, Bob Stevens, who has been at my side—dependable, loving and caring. I want to thank my three children, Lisa, Eric and Gina; my mother, Grace McFadden; and my twin sister, Gracie Lee, for their prayers and moral support.

Mary J. Stevens

Acknowledgements

My deepest gratitude to the many fantastic doctors, both named and unnamed, who have cared for me over the years, because without them, I would not be here today.

Heartfelt thanks to the seven people described in this book, who shared an important part of their lives with us, for the sole purpose of helping others.

Many thanks to my devoted editor, Joan West, who worked tirelessly to encourage me to bring my story to life. In addition, thanks to Lois Bennett, Joan's partner, for her input and support.

My thanks to Mark Newhouse, who encouraged me and introduced me to Joan.

I definitely want to thank a great, national organization known as the PNA, the Pituitary Network Association, and its chairman, Robert Knutzen, for allowing us to use material from their resource books and magazines. This huge organization offers support groups for patients and relatives of people with pituitary problems. Through their books, newsletters, national conferences and support groups, the PNA reaches not only people experiencing pituitary problems, but also hospitals, universities and medical centers. It exists for the sole purpose of helping each individual to improve, heal and recover. PNA desires to increase awareness of the vast medical problems that often accompany pituitary disease.

Mary J. Stevens

CONTENTS

Mary J. Stevens

Chapter 1

You Need Sex!

"You need sex! That would solve your whole problem."

I was stunned. This couldn't be happening to me, Sister Leah Patrice, a Catholic nun of the order of the Sisters of St. Joseph. Humiliated, I stood in the doctor's examining room, partially disrobed and feeling vulnerable.

Many years of ill health, accompanied by unceasing fatigue had brought me to that devastating moment. During the mid-1950's, when I was in my early twenties, my voice had begun changing, taking on a deeper, hollow-sounding quality. Sometimes, I seemed to be mimicking Lauren Bacall, the movie star; yet, due to the gradual onset, I was unaware that my throat muscles were actually thickening.

For two years prior to my humiliating experience in the doctor's examining room, I had discussed my physical symptoms with many other doctors. I had complained about the violent headaches, the nausea and the dizziness deep inside my head, accompanied by flashing colored lights coming at me from a distance, then spreading, becoming larger, and disappearing. Yet, no doctor ever recommended that I have neurological tests, or any other kind performed. My diagnosis had consistently been that I had "the flu."

Finally, my superior at the convent recommended that I have a complete physical examination from Doctor X, a local doctor, who also came highly recommended by several other people. In my initial discussion with Doctor X, I informed him of my health issues, including the four-year cessation of my menstrual cycle, the migraine headaches and the flashing lights, dizziness, nausea and constant fatigue.

Perhaps, my expectations were too high; yet, this time, I thought my health problems might actually be resolved. Instead, I had the infuriating diagnosis of "You need sex." This man, who had taken the Hippocratic Oath, continued to insult me.

"Your lifestyle is too rigorous," he said. "You need to relax, but your real problem is that you need sex, and I can help you with that."

As he talked, he quickly gave me an injection.

I had nearly stopped listening until the shock of the needle brought me back to attention.

"What is the purpose of the shot you just gave me?" I asked.

"Testosterone. It's a male hormone that may correct your problem."

With my head spinning, I heard the rasping sound of his voice still rambling.

"You can come to my house and swim in my indoor pool, and I will take care of you. I'll teach you to relax. Don't bother bringing a bathing suit," he added. "My place is totally private."

"Absolutely not," I stammered, shocked at his proposal. "I can't believe you are saying this to me. I'm a nun."

I must be in a dream. How can a doctor be talking to me like this? Why?

My quick refusal of his offer to help me brought a fast response.

"You're going to end up in a mental institution. You need a psychiatrist," he shouted. "You'll be in a psychiatric ward within a year with your emotional problems. Your symptoms are all in your head."

Angry and upset, his words still ringing in my ears, I quickly dressed and stoically left the consulting room, vowing I would never return.

At that time, nuns were not allowed to leave the convent alone and one of my associates, Sister Mary Benedict, sat patiently in the waiting room. You can imagine her questioning look, when I came rushing out and said, "Come on, Sister. We're through here."

I felt too embarrassed and distraught to tell anyone what the doctor had said. Today, I would respond differently, but in the late fifties, I believed this was my only option. For days, I prayed to the Lord, asking Him for guidance through His Holy Spirit.

God, you called me to this special vocation. You must have a special plan for me. I know because you always take care of me. God, I really need your help right now.

Shortly after Doctor X's upsetting outburst at me, Sister Mary Benedict and I took a trip to our mother house at Nazareth, Michigan, just outside of Kalamazoo. On the way, we stopped at Borgess Hospital. One of my classmates, Sister Mary Barbara, who had been a nurse before entering the convent, was in charge of the psychiatric ward.

I chose not to tell Sister Mary Barbara about my emotional state. With the doctor's ominous words echoing in my mind, *"You're going to end up in a mental institution,"* I asked Sister to take us on a tour of the psych ward, using the ploy that I'd like to see where she worked. As we strolled through the halls, I looked into the padded locked rooms, where some of the patients seemed to be normal, while others cowered in corners, and still others appeared to be in another world.

"There is very little furniture in most of the rooms because we don't want the patients to hurt themselves," Sister Mary Barbara remarked.

I saw that some of the rooms had no furniture at all, just built-in beds. Realizing that some of the patients appeared to be quite normal, while others seemed weird to me, I began to personalize the situation.

Will this be me in the future? Was that doctor right in his prediction?

We thanked Sister Mary Barbara, and once outside the hospital, I began to cry. I felt scared and so alone. Sister Mary Benedict became concerned and wanted to know why I was crying.

"That psych ward really bothered me," I said. "All those people in there; can their problems ever be resolved? It's so sad!"

As we quietly walked to our car in the parking lot, I forced myself to calm down. *God has always been at my side. He will be there to help me. I know it, and I firmly believe in Him. I trust and walk with God!*

Sister Mary Benedict and I immediately drove to the mother house at Nazareth, where she took off to visit with some friends, while I quickly went to the chapel to pray. I loved the coolness, the darkness and the beauty of that little chapel. I sat down to meditate, but my thoughts began to roam back to the days of my childhood.

Chapter 2

Growing Up as a Twin

On May 7, 1934 at seven minutes past seven in the evening, I entered this world and three minutes later, my sister, Gracie Lee, appeared. We often wondered whether I, Mary Jane McFadden, was destined to arrive first, or were we just playing around in the womb and by the luck of the draw, I pushed my way out first.

Lee and I were each born with a thin veil of skin over our faces. Someone told our mother that the veil, or caul, was a sign of good luck. As the story goes, ship captains often wanted to have it on board their vessels to bring them good luck at sea. In keeping with the way unusual memorabilia is often preserved, our family doctor, Dr. Jordan, placed the veils in a jar with a liquid solution and advised our parents to keep it. When we were a little older, it became an object of teasing from our brothers, who joked that the veil of skin should never have been removed, especially, if one of us had just tattled on them.

Neither of us showed any of our mother's German or French traits of dark hair and dark skin tones. Mother's irritation surfaced, when strangers asked whether her nearly bald twins with strawberry blond fuzz covering their heads were adopted. She soon grew tired of explaining that her babies looked like their Irish father, Dixon McFadden.

As youngsters, we all called my twin sister, Lee, because it was easier for us to pronounce than Gracie. She and I enjoyed being twins, even thinking of ourselves as "mirror" twins, since I favored my right hand, while Lee always used her left hand. We often were chosen to lead parades or to perform the Irish jig on

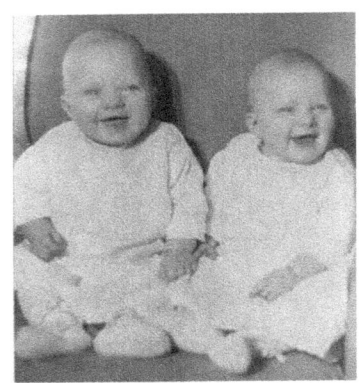

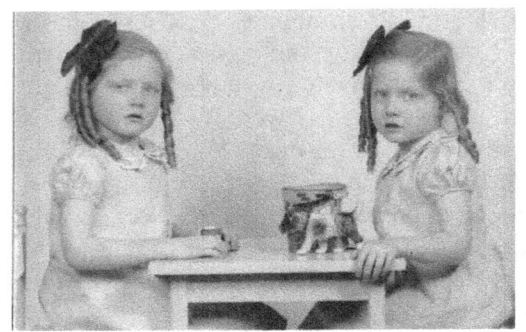

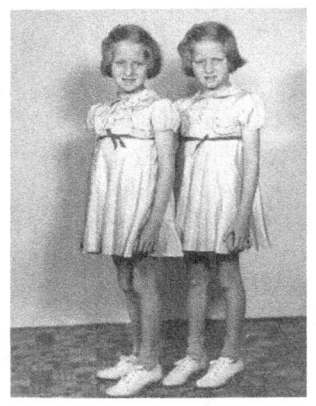

Identical Twins

stage for Saint Patrick's Day, which, of course, pleased our Irish daddy. Teachers often placed us at the head of the line to help quickly identify where their class lines began. It was really special when we were sent together on errands to upper grade classes, so our teacher could "show the twins off."

"Do you ever wake up and think you are your sister and your sister is you?" This heads the list of silly questions adults often asked us. Then there was, "Don't you hate sharing everything, even your birthdays?"

"What is it like not to share?" came our response.

We did all the things you might see twins do in the movies. We talked at the same time, both saying the same thing, or one would start a sentence and the other finish it. We frequently felt each other's mood or pain, and when one twin got hurt, we both cried. Some of the perks associated with being identical twins were fun, such as getting into the movies free.

There were five children in our family, including Jim and Dick, our older brothers, and a younger sister named Patricia. At times, Lee and I laughed through our tears over skinned knees and elbows, when our confused brothers resorted to calling us "Sis" or "Sissie," as they tried to remember who owned the scar.

Being a twin was fun, especially when we went shopping. Our parents bought two of everything. If Lee chose one dress and I chose another, they usually bought two of each. Sometimes, it meant driving from Sears or Federals Department Store in Highland Park to Sears or Federals in Ferndale in order to get a matching dress or coat.

I was a bit more tomboyish than my twin. Often, I climbed trees and rode my brother Dick's motorbike, where-as my twin was interested in other activities. For our birthdays, we each had our own cake, and the presents were always identical–just like we were. Everything came in twos.

During elementary school, our teachers and friends must have wondered about our family. While most children have only two grandmas, we had the usual two plus the cleaning women our dad hired and who we were instructed to call "Grandma." Our dad would hire these "grandmas" and our mother would fire them. There were others, but I only remember Grandma Moses and Grandma Mona. Grandma Mona stayed the longest. I don't know why. She was the one who put our dresses on backward and combed our hair funny. Then Mom took over the household by herself.

When I was about eight or nine-years-old, I fell at school and smashed my front teeth on a metal pipe. Lee and I both felt excruciating pain. Someone called my dad and he rushed me to the dental office. My upper permanent front teeth were all broken. I often thank my dad for his foresight. He insisted the teeth be capped immediately. The pain was bad enough, but the look of broken teeth would have been terrible.

I was hit with a hardball around the same age, when a line drive at a baseball game pummeled my right breast. It became painful and swollen. I had to endure annual biopsies for three years, checking for cancer. After the third biopsy, thankfully, the swelling and pain gradually subsided.

Lee and I had begun swimming lessons with the "Y" at Nolan Junior High, but I had to quit after the first two lessons. It was time for my first biopsy and I had to enter the hospital. I was discharged by the time of Lee's graduation ceremony, and my parents and I watched as Lee passed the first phase of swimming tests and received her certificate. The instructor had suggested that I put on a bathing suit to watch. After Lee did her floats, swam the length of the pool, then dived in and swam underwater, everyone clapped.

"Anything Lee can do, I can do, too. We're twins." I jumped into the water, passed all the tests, and received my certificate for accomplishment, too.

Shortly before Christmas, when we were to have school pictures taken for the spring yearbook, I developed a large cold sore on my lip. Instead of using my picture with this blemish, we submitted two pictures of Lee–both the same picture. It was our secret, still teachers and classmates found differences between us in the pictures, positive they could tell us apart!

Throughout our Catholic schooling, I participated in sports programs at lunch hour, attended meditation groups after school, and always tried to attend daily Mass. I had a great love for my God and had developed a great trust in His Providence. This no doubt stemmed from my parents, who exhibited strong faith in their God and from the dedicated teachers (Sisters) who seemed to walk so close to God.

Although, Lee and I often attended different functions and classes, arriving at school at St. Rita's High School at different times, when we eventually got together, we invariably found that we were dressed alike. One of us had arisen earlier, gotten dressed and left before the other was up, but we still selected the same clothing. It just happened.

Over the next several years, I experienced a lot of pain in my lower abdomen. A physical check-up with our family doctor, Dr. Jordon, produced no positive results. The doctor said it was "probably the flu." When I walked hunched over, the pain lessened, but it periodically reappeared, getting worse, as the years went by.

When I was sixteen, both Lee and I worked at Kresge's dime store. Lee worked toward the back of the store on the hardware counter, and I sold cosmetics up front. One day, I doubled up in pain, falling to the floor. I had read about how painful cancer could be and was sure that it might be causing my pain.

I prayed to God with great emotion.

God, please don't let me die. If I survive and live, I will immediately join the convent.

I had always admired the nun's dedication to God and the great spiritual life they must have with God. They often told me that perhaps He was calling me to the religious life. It made me wonder, if I had a vocation, a calling to be a nun.

All this went through my mind, as I thought I was going to die. I hurt so badly. Lee felt my pain and came running to the front of the store yelling for help.

Since calling 911 for an emergency was still years away, the store manager called my dad. Dad called Dr. Jordon, who instructed that I should be packed in ice and driven to the hospital as quickly as possible. Fortunately for me, my dad, an office manager for an insurance company, worked only five miles away. He arrived quickly and the store manager, who had seen to it that I was packed in ice, helped me into the car and my dad rushed me to the hospital. I'm sure he broke a few speed limits. My appendix had ruptured and I was rushed into the operating room for an emergency appendectomy. Thanks to my sister, the quick thinking store manager and my dad, I survived. It was February 14, 1951. Happy Valentine's Day!

Immediately upon recovery, I began to make plans to enter the convent of the Sisters of St. Joseph. I kept my word with God.

Chapter 3

Convent Life

The Sisters of St. Joseph is a religious order dedicated to serving God through teaching and nursing. On July 1, 1951, I entered the Convent located in Nazareth, Michigan. I entered, as a postulant, preparing for religious life. The Class of 1951 began its new lifestyle amid excitement and anticipation, yet completely unaware of what the future held.

At that time, I weighed one hundred pounds and stood five-feet-five-inches tall. Homesickness hit me hard. I missed my parents and my brothers and sisters, especially Lee.

As a postulant, my first "lesson" was an introduction to the schedule of convent living and the rules and regulations that had become a part of my new life. Chores, something new for me, were assigned.

My immaturity surfaced, as I learned about cleaning, scrubbing and washing clothes, even my own socks. I had never cleaned a whole house or, for that matter, not even a room. My mother had never wanted us to make our own beds. That was her job, she said, preferring to converse with us in the mornings, rather than saddling us with housework. Evenings, we children washed or dried dishes, but that was the extent of our household chores.

Reading, working on school projects, practicing music lessons, playing outside and becoming involved in after-school activities were all more important to Mom than having us do housework. All five children were required to take some form of music lessons for enrichment. Lee and I chose lessons on the Hawaiian guitar and for the next eight years, daily practice—required by our parents and teachers—became part of our lives.

19

My ineptness at cleaning a refectory, scrubbing and buffing stairs and hallways, and performing all the other cleaning tasks highlighted my lack of experience in manual labor. Never had I experienced such exertion before, and I felt a level of exhaustion that was totally new to me.

Convent living followed a rigorous and highly structured daily schedule. The sound of a bell signaled us to rise in silence at five o'clock in the morning and gather in the chapel twenty minutes later. There, we participated in morning prayers and meditation, followed by worship at Mass.

After breakfast, each sister performed her assigned chores and then attended both educational and religious classes. Spiritual reading was common during meals, but on Sundays, and occasionally on one or two other days during the week, conversation would be allowed at dinner. Regulations were less rigorously enforced when on mission for a teaching assignment.

Conversation could take place at meals on special days, such as Christmas, Easter, Memorial Day, New Year's Day, Thanksgiving, the Fourth of July and, of course, St. Joseph's Day. Those were days of celebration; but after meals, continuous quiet time ensued for more prayer, reflections or study.

If we chose to, we could converse for one hour each afternoon in the recreation room of the convent. Afterward, we gathered in the chapel for Vespers and meditation, concluding with the rosary.

After dinner and before evening prayers, another hour was set aside for conversation; however, this time, participation was a requirement, not an option. By nine o'clock, each sister retired in quiet and solitude to her room. The sisters always observed silence throughout the convent, except in the refectory, recreation room and outdoors, when allowed. Silence could be broken for an emergency–the only reason to break the rule.

In September, 1951, accelerated classes began; so I was able to graduate from high school and begin college immediately. Throughout these formative months in the convent, Mother Leonella, the Novice Mistress, constantly stressed that we must mix with everyone. Absolutely no particular friendships were allowed. Superiors monitored any signs of lesbianism and, if found, ordered the individual to leave the convent at once. I observed these precepts religiously and spent my years in the convent basically alone, with no confidante close enough to discuss, or be aware of, my personal problems.

Conversations among the sisters had to be uplifting, never negative. Jokingly, one sister might say, "Think the rain will hurt the rhubarb?" and another sister would reply, "Not if it's in the cellar in cans."

We often walked outside during good weather and stopped by the cemetery to pray for our deceased nuns and to enjoy the beautiful grounds. I frequently walked the grounds, praying the rosary, or I sat outside to study.

Time moved swiftly during the six-month postulancy, and soon came the exciting moment of dedication. My family attended for this spiritual and emotional experience. Each postulant walked down the aisle in the chapel as a bride, requesting the right to become a Sister of Saint Joseph, as a novice.

I left the chapel as Mary Jane McFadden. Upon returning, dressed as a Sister of Saint Joseph, I knelt before the bishop at the altar and was given the name I had requested, Sister Leah Patrice.

Since I always called my twin, Lee, the closest religious name acceptable was Leah and Patrice for my other sister, Patricia. I made the choice to leave behind everything of the world and live a religious life, as I had promised God on Valentine's Day. I truly expected that I would live the rest of my life as a nun.

The next period of my new life, the novitiate, was structured around prayer, work, dedication, education and training. The novice mistress, Mother Leonella, displayed exceptional understanding and kindness. I came to respect and love her dearly.

More and more, I began to experience extreme fatigue, near exhaustion. My body required rest or long periods of sleep after any exertion. I often fell asleep in the chapel or during my studies, making it difficult to concentrate on my task.

Severe migraine headaches along with nausea and dizziness

nearly overwhelmed me at times, especially when accompanied by excessive sweating and lack of appetite. Flashing colored lights creating an element of disorientation swirled toward me during both waking hours and sleep.

I loved the quiet, cool temperatures and the darkness of the chapel. Bright lights often hurt my eyes, causing optometrists to indicate that the cups in my eyes were too large, which could be an indicator for the future development of glaucoma. But my medical doctors continued to diagnose me as having "the flu."

Mother Leonella, frequently interrupted my work to send me to the chapel to pray, allowing me to rest. She changed my work assignments and lightened my workload, so I wouldn't be overly tired.

During nice weather, I enjoyed my outside work-station, sweeping the grotto. I'm sure she thought the sun and air would invigorate me; but the headaches, flashes of light, nausea and dizziness continued, along with an erratic menstrual cycle, which had started about age fourteen, much later than my sister.

Mother Leonella was an older nun, who appeared in touch with the Lord at all times. She was such a saintly person that when she spoke of loving Him, her whole face beamed, radiating His love. Her eyes shone and sometimes, she choked up, having great difficulty getting out the words that she wanted to say about the greatness of the Lord. Although I knew she walked hand-in-hand with God, it was only later that I learned that people from the local community often came to speak with her to seek her spiritual counsel.

My health problems continued. Mother Leonella thought that, if I gained weight, my problems would be solved. Five-feet-five-inches tall and weighing in at one hundred pounds was thin. Gaining weight would definitely be a sign of happiness and belonging and should make me feel better, she thought. Eating more at mealtimes was an impossible task for me, so Mother Leonella had a medication prescribed for me to take one hour prior to meals. Unfortunately, rather than increasing my appetite, it made me so nauseous, I couldn't eat at all.

Her next remedy came in the form of drinking eggnog and eating a couple of cookies in the afternoon. To me, the eggnogs tasted slimy and gagged me, but I forced them down. The nuns in the kitchen prepared the drinks and varied the flavors to make them more palatable. I had everything from chocolate or peach to lemon, vanilla and apricot. Still, I did not gain weight.

Adding to the eggnogs, the novice mistress then ordered me to take two vitamins daily along with twelve yeast tablets, which I did for the next several months, but with no change in results. The fatigue continued.

"I don't want to offend you, but are you sure you aren't Pinocchio? I swear your nose is growing," one of my classmates commented. She was serious.

My parents suggested that I loosen the headpiece around my face. They thought it pushed my face outward, making my features look larger. The headgear had to be worn snug to the face; nothing could be done to change that. Later, I learned that my parents had put towels around Lee's hair to see if we still looked alike.

In reality, facial growth changes were happening to me, but so gradually, I didn't recognize the problem. Nuns don't analyze themselves before mirrors.

The caps that had been put on my front teeth years ago were connected together. Now, at age seventeen, the permanent bridge on my front teeth began to break and crack. I had to visit a dentist to have the bridgework redone.

The severe migraine headaches, dizziness and nausea continued. At times, I had difficulty walking and now, I also had difficulty concentrating on my studies; yet, my diagnosis remained the same: I had "the flu."

My parents began to wonder what was wrong with me because Lee felt ill; yet, there was nothing wrong with her. It had to be related to me, they thought. I'm sure they were extremely worried, but tried not to show it. Thank God, after being separated for a period of time, Lee, who had requested that she be called Gracie, no longer felt my pain and emotions.

Rules regarding visits from our relatives were quite strict. They could visit only once a month, on the second or third Sunday afternoon, and only from one o'clock to four o'clock,

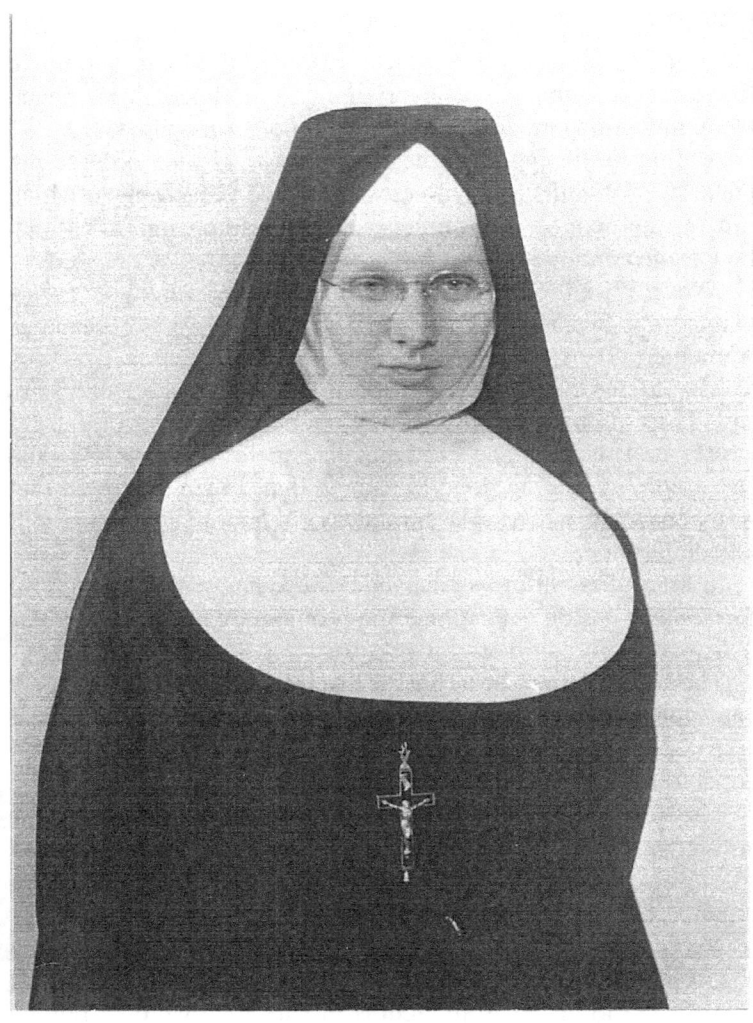

Sister Leah Patrice (McFadden), S.S.J., professing her final vows with the Sisters of St. Joseph, Nazareth, Michigan. Notice the larger bottom lip, the beginning of a hang lip and the larger nose; the wider jowl had not yet started.

and never during Lent or Advent. We were allowed to make phone calls only in emergency situations. Home visitation was not allowed, and we could not attend weddings or baptisms. We could attend funerals, but only for the immediate family. We were permitted to receive letters from our families; however all mail going out and coming in was censored.

We did not have the freedom to turn on a radio or television or even read the newspaper. With the superior's permission, we were allowed to view some educational shows, such as the talk shows of Bishop Sheen; however, the convent schedule was rigorously enforced. When it was time for prayer, the television was turned off, even if the show we were watching wasn't over.

When teaching, we were allowed to attend PTA functions and any programs put on by the students. These exceptions were approved and a part of our teaching careers.

During my two year novitiate, my thyroid levels were tested at a nearby hospital. The results fell within the normal range. The doctor, aware of my continued headaches and extreme sensitivity to light, pronounced a somewhat different diagnosis this time.

"Since there is nothing physically wrong with you, you must be having a severe emotional problem," he said. "Perhaps, the lifestyle is too strenuous for you and you don't belong in the convent."

Mother Leonella agreed to the first part of this diagnosis, but not the second.

"Your emotional problem must be caused because you miss your twin sister," she said. "This is a perfectly normal reaction and, therefore, *not* a reason to leave the convent."

Finally, January of 1953 arrived and my classmates and I walked down the aisle and requested to profess our vows before the community of nuns and the bishop, the prelate of the church. Individually, we each pronounced our temporary vows of poverty, chastity and obedience, seeking to be members of the Sisters of Saint Joseph.

We were then given our assignments, our missions. Mine was teaching at a parish school. I enjoyed teaching children, working with choral groups, teaching catechetical classes, and in some parishes, helping with cleaning and decorating the altar with bouquets of flowers.

The three years went by quickly, and suddenly, it was time for final vows. There still had been no relief found for my headaches, which sometimes affected only one side of my head and other times were deep-seated, encompassing the whole area of my head. Flashing colored lights found me in my sleep as well as during waking hours. Fatigue, nausea, dizziness inside my head–all these things continually plagued me. I questioned whether it was emotional, as the doctor suggested or could it still be something physical? There were no ready answers.

Each year, the sisters attended a one-week retreat and a one-day retreat was added on the last Sunday of each month. Before taking our final vows, we attended a special retreat for prayer and reflection.

Suddenly, my rambling thoughts were interrupted, as the rest of the community of nuns arrived in the chapel for afternoon vespers, meditation and rosary and, together, we worshiped our Lord.

But my thoughts repeatedly refocused on the psychiatric ward I had just seen at Borgess Hospital. I began to pray in earnest.

God, I am so worried. I do not believe You would let this happen to me. I trust in Your Providence. I beg You to give me Your guidance and Your direction.

After prayers, I dined with the Sisters at the Mother House and then returned to the convent, feeling so upset, so disturbed, and the only one I could turn to was God. I had never felt so alone.

When I took my final vows, my family again was there to share this time of dedication and reflection.

Once again, my classmates and I approached the altar before the congregation of the sisters and the bishop, each to profess our final vows of poverty, chastity and obedience. I truly believed I had made my commitment to God for life.

Chapter 4

My Teaching Career

Throughout my teaching career, I remained unaware that facial changes and other distortions were taking place in my body. Perhaps the old maxim, "hindsight is 20/20," would fit here. My hair had begun to grow rapidly with the new growth coming in coarse and thick. My teeth and jaw had protruded and my nose increased in size, especially on one side. Enlarged lips with a hang lip, coarser, oily skin with rashes, and enlargement of the tongue, all resulted in a considerable change in my appearance. I also experienced dry mouth and the increased hair growth spread from my face to all parts of my body.

Still another more drastic change took place about the time I turned twenty-six; my menstrual cycle began again. I felt a great relief. With precision, every four weeks on a Friday morning at seven a.m., it was there–my monthly visitor. This came as a complete surprise to me. It had never been so regular before.

Once again, the bridge on my upper front teeth began to crack, forcing me to start another dental regimen to have a new bridge installed on those same teeth.

As I had done all my adult life, I continually prayed for guidance from the Lord. I stayed extremely busy with my work assignments along with my personal life of prayer and worship of my God. By the 1960s, the migraine headaches and nausea had slowed down for which I thanked a kind and gracious God.

I still felt an ongoing dizziness and pressure way inside of my head, behind my eyes. I never felt quite right, but could not pinpoint the real problem. Night driving became especially tenuous, as my sensitivity to light remained with me. My fatigue problems worsened, as the physical changes increased. On many occasions, I had to ask permission to retire early. My frustrations mounted, since I really didn't understand what type of curse could have attacked my body.

My first teaching assignment was at a nearby grade school.

"You should not fast during Advent and Lent," the pastor of the church and school told me. "We want our teachers to be healthy, and I don't want to have to hire a substitute teacher for you."

Each parish school I went to after that must have heard the word, because I received the same admonition each year. Although I was five-feet-five-inches tall, I weighed only around one hundred pounds, which apparently caused them all to presume that I also lacked energy. Unfortunately, their presumption was correct. I still tired easily, required extra rest, and continually had severe headaches.

At one of the small schools, where I taught, space was so limited that the music teacher gave piano lessons in the living room of the convent. When I experienced one of my "flu" spells with migraines, the teacher kindly rescheduled her students for a couple of days, so I could enjoy excellent piano music. I was so ill, I never even heard them, but it was sweet of her to think of me.

I always taught in the elementary schools, serving grades one through eight. Usually, I taught the upper elementary classes, specializing in English literature and English usage. I also taught other subjects, such as religion, music and art. At times, I had fun directing choral groups or choirs.

With our teaching duties on hold, summers usually brought several invitations for the Sisters of Saint Joseph to use someone's cottage for boating and recreation. Of course, it was always done with discretion and privacy. At one cottage, a couple of us got into a rowboat and rowed out into the middle of the lake to relax and enjoy the view. The lapping of the water against the boat lulled us into a relaxed state, and we didn't pay much attention to the darkening sky, as it became more and more threatening.

"Come in, right away. A severe storm warning has been issued," the gentleman, who owned the cottage, yelled from the shoreline.

Immediately, two of the nuns began rowing, but the boat felt sluggish and it was slow going. Finally, we arrived at the shore.

"Next time, pull up the anchor. It would make it a lot easier to row," the owner said.

We had forgotten that we had dropped anchor. We felt so dumb, but had a good laugh over it anyway.

Often, when we visited a cottage, I was the one who drove the motorboat at high speed around the lake with all the sisters' veils flying.

One time, we had been assigned a teaching mission at a parish, where we had been warned that proper decorum was particularly important, because many of the residents were not friendly toward Catholics and nuns. When we nuns arrived and stepped out of the car, the parish priest welcomed us. He introduced us to a visiting non-English speaking Mexican priest, who was there for the migrant workers.

Leaving our luggage in the car, the local priest took us and his visitor down to the river front to show us his motorboat. Imagine our surprise, when he stripped down to his bathing suit.

Apparently, my reputation preceded me, for the priest asked me to take the controls, while he water-skied. I had never steered a boat pulling a water-skier before, let alone a priest, let alone a priest in his bathing suit!

"I don't get a chance to water-ski very often," he said. "Keep it at full speed."

Racing up and down the river at full speed with two nuns in the boat, a Mexican priest, who didn't speak English, and with a priest in a bathing suit skimming over the water behind us, was a new experience for me. The river curved and narrowed, so moving at full speed, I had to turn the boat around quickly at breakneck speed and head back up the river until it narrowed again. After several trips up and down the river, the wake of the boat caused some huge logs to float out toward the middle of the river, coming downstream straight toward the boat.

Still going full speed, with me dodging the logs and the water-skiing priest jumping over the logs, I steered too close to the steep shoreline. Suddenly, the boat tipped on its side. We held on for dear life, speeding along sideways on the bank of the river. I was really scared, terrified that we might flip over. I had no command over that boat.

"Jesus, Mary, Joseph," one of the nuns yelled over and over.

The Mexican priest continually prayed aloud in Spanish, blessing himself all the while. The other sister laughed, but looked petrified. She was not alone; I, too, was petrified.

Finally, the riverbed curved, the boat straightened out and we leveled off into the water, bringing us back into the center of the river. I quickly turned the boat around, slowed down and docked. The water-skiing priest had slipped off his ski board into the water without injury. That ride was definitely over. We never did it again.

With that venture, we knew the townspeople must surely be aware that we had arrived in town. So much for decorum!

Later that day, Sister Dorothy Marie and I went to a local grocery store to stock up the convent pantry. As we placed our food selections on the counter for the cashier to ring up, she took each item, put it into another basket and ordered a stock boy to put the items back on the shelf.

"Move out, please! Make room for the next customer," she ordered.

Rather than cause a scene, we left the store and had our local housekeeper buy the groceries for us. Other than having been called a witch a few times, this was my first taste of discrimination. I must say, I did not like it.

We had a very successful year opening the new school. By mid-year, my children's choir was singing beautifully. We practiced during Lent for a great Easter celebration at Mass. I knew the congregation would be impressed with the students' accomplishments, when their lovely voices sang the Latin Mass.

Unfortunately, the week before Easter, heavy, beating rainstorms arrived, turning the rural roads into soggy mud and making them impassable for cars or trucks. All the schools were closed. I never expected my choir students to show up for the Easter celebration of Mass.

"The people will come," the parish priest kept saying.

What a shocking surprise. The farmers covered their tractor lifts with cloth, carried their children in the lifts and came across the fields in their tractors–coming to worship God on Easter Sunday. The small country church was filled to capacity. What beautiful faith. The choir performed perfectly, and I was so proud of them. That Easter was a day of thanksgiving.

Many of the people in the small town had become quite friendly by the time the school year ended, so some changes did occur. As we were leaving in June, many of the townspeople commented, "Hope to see you ladies next September."

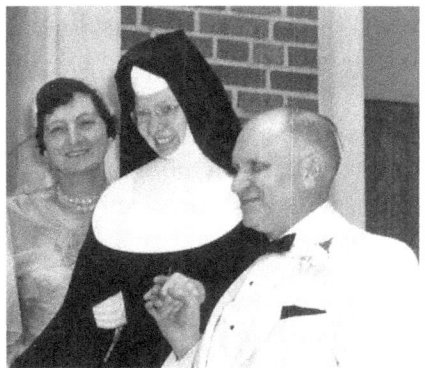

June 1960, Sister Leah Patrice, S.S.J., standing on the front steps of the convent with my mother and father, Grace and Dixon McFadden. Dad stood below me on the sidewalk. I was five feet five inches tall and Dad was five-foot-eleven. I never grew taller with acromegaly—some people do.

31

I still did not have my college degree, so each summer, I took a condensed college class, attended summer school, and then took another condensed college class at Nazareth, the Mother House.

One September in the early 1960s, my assignment took me to the seventh grade in a wealthy parish. I met Sister Mary Patrick, an inner-city teacher in Detroit. Together, we worked out a student exchange program. This allowed our students to reach out and meet other children, so they could understand more about children and families of different ethnic backgrounds and incomes. My students were all white, mostly upper income. Her students were Hispanic, white and black, mostly lower income.

We prepared the children by having discussions on values, educational and job opportunities, and the understanding that poor is not synonymous with dirty. Parents signed authorization slips, and the program began.

We bussed half of my students to the inner-city school, and the other half became involved in programs to welcome students from the Detroit school. This included inviting the students to their homes for lunch with interesting results.

The students were especially surprised at the common behavior of their mothers. One of our students, whose father was an attorney, was surprised when she brought a visitor home for lunch. Her mother wanted to make a good impression, so she put a tablecloth and a bouquet of fresh-cut flowers on the kitchen table. She served the lunch in courses, which she had never done before–soup first, then a sandwich, followed by desert.

"My lunch is never like this. My mother went overboard to make this luncheon special for you," the student commented to the visiting student on the way back to school.

During our discussions following the student-exchange day, another student had a similar comment. She visited at an inner-city home. When they got to the house, the mother had a tablecloth on the table and served them soup, followed by a hot dog and then cake. The Detroit girl was quite surprised.

"We don't put tablecloths on for dinner, let alone lunch. My mother did this specially for you."

When washing up for lunch, one of the suburban girls noticed that the water from the bathroom sink drained into a bucket, which was emptied into the toilet. The inner-city girl's father had died and her mother could not afford a plumber to fix the sink. A friendship developed between the girls over a few months and the suburban family offered to do repairs for the Detroit family. Many similar events happened, as a result of that student exchange. The children became pen pals, visited each other, and exchanged gifts.

The overall experience enriched all the students involved. Sister Mary Patrick was pleased with her students' comments, one of which was, "If I stay in school and get a good education, I could possibly have a lifestyle like the kids in the suburbs."

It was experiences like this one that make me love teaching.

Chapter 5

A Difficult Decision

"Perhaps God did call you to this vocation, but now He may have other plans for you," a spiritual advisor suggested.

Was she right? Was it time for me to leave the convent? I was here because I loved God and wanted to serve him in the best way possible; but it had to be His way, not mine.

"Since doctors indicate that your health problems are really emotional problems, perhaps this is a direct message from God to you that you really don't belong in the convent," another spiritual advisor had said.

Was He using this means of directing me to the understanding that this portion of my life had served His purpose, and now I should move on?

"Just because you are considered an excellent teacher, doesn't mean you should stay on as a nun. Good teachers are needed everywhere," I was told.

Was serving by teaching to be my mission, now?

I left for my yearly seven day retreat at the Mother House during Christmas vacation in 1963, my mind in turmoil. For several years, I had heard these types of statements from spiritual counselors. Were they right? Was mine just an emotional problem or, too awful to contemplate, was it a psychiatric problem? Had Doctor X been right that I might end up in a mental institution? I just didn't know.

During the retreat, I prayed extensively over this momentous decision. I tried to be logical and analyze my health problems through the fifty's and now, still into the sixty's. The problems never seemed to disappear. What if the advisors were right and God did call me to the convent, but now He is directing me to go somewhere else?

I wished that God would knock me in the head and let me know what to do. After all, he did knock St. Paul to the ground and blinded him to get His message across. The retreat was over and I remained undecided, but back at the convent, I realized that I couldn't put it off any longer. God wasn't going to knock me to the ground. I had to do it myself and, difficult as it was, I had to do it now.

In January of 1964, I sent a petition/request through the Reverend Mother to the Holy Father in Rome to be dispensed from my final vows.

While waiting for a reply from Rome, the Reverend Mother asked me not to tell any of the sisters that I was leaving. I complied with her wishes and remained silent, as I went about preparing to leave the convent, my home for the past thirteen years.

Most of the sisters kept their hair cut very short under the habit and I had done this also. Now, I let my hair grow long, but kept it totally hidden by the habit. As it grew, my anxiety over my decision grew. As I slowly put my longer and longer hair up under my habit in a pony tail, the reality of what I was doing caused me great concern.

I would be thirty-years-old. How would I function in the real world after thirteen years of living in a convent and having all the daily necessities taken care of for me? How would I find a job, deal with personal finances, make all the large and small decisions that living out in the world would entail?

Was my decision really God's message to me? Plagued as I was with questions and still no direct answer as to what to do, I spent hours in prayer in the small convent chapel, asking God to guide me.

God! Please give me guidance and strength and give me peace of mind!

The school year came to an end and I returned to the Mother House at Nazareth to continue to take the college classes that I needed for my degree.

The Mother Superior received the dispensation in late July 1964 and asked me if I wanted to accept or reject it. Fear of the unknown had engulfed me during the months that I waited for my dispensation. Fear sways so many decisions. Sometimes, it is easier to just accept the status quo, which in some ways, I longed to do.

I prayed, once again, that God would send His Spirit to lead me in the right direction.

I accepted the dispensation. In August 1964, I left the convent. After thirteen years, I was no longer a Sister of St. Joseph.

Chapter 6

Home Again

My parents were not surprised when I notified them that I would be coming home. Over the years, they had sensed that something was wrong, but they did not know what it could be. Were they disappointed? Probably. But they never voiced it.

The first week of August, some of the sisters were headed to St. Anne's Convent in Detroit for their next teaching assignment, and I rode into Detroit with them, sitting in silence. I had followed the Reverend Mother's request that I tell no one; so they didn't know I was leaving. I realized that I had spent almost half of my life in the convent, protected, secluded, and alone. Now the Spirit guided me into a whole new direction. So scary and so frightening! It was really happening. I was really leaving the convent.

On the drive to Detroit, I watched the landscape speed by, yet time seemed to move so slowly. I prayed asking God to continually guide me through this time of transition.

Please give me direction, give me help and especially give me strength.

I remained at St. Anne's Convent for a few hours waiting for my parents to pick me up. The refrain continued to run through my mind: *I have no job, no credit, no clothes, and absolutely no idea of what my new path will be.*

I had asked my mother to bring some of her clothes, since I had nothing to wear. My twin, Gracie was married several years before, and lived in a southwestern suburb of Detroit with her husband and two small boys (one just eight months old), so borrowing some of her clothes was not an option. My mom was much shorter than I and her shoe size much smaller. She brought a pair of sandals for me so I could be comfortable without pinched toes on the way home.

When my parents arrived, I changed into the less than fashion-fitting clothes my mother had provided and we began the drive home. Excitement showed in my parents' voices as they asked question after question: *What are your plans? What kind of help do you need? How do you feel?* I, in turn asked a million questions about them and about my brothers and sisters and their families.

As soon as we got home, I excitedly called my twin sister for the first time in thirteen years. We talked for a long time, interrupting each other constantly. Gracie invited me to visit her once I got settled into a job and a routine. Priorities had to come first.

Now came a much needed haircut and styling. The beautician commented that my hair was so thick that she could use me in hair shows, and later did just that. Then, Mom and I had fun shopping. I needed everything—underwear, clothing, coats, and shoes. I also had to establish credit of my own, since I had no money. Thirty years old and I'd never had a credit card! Dad cosigned for the credit cards, and I bought everything I needed for fall and early winter, even a winter coat.

We had to strip the manikins in some of the store windows in order to get my size. When we left those stores, Mom and I gazed at the store fronts and laughed.

"When I see naked manikins," she would say, "I know Mary must have visited that store." We had fun.

That evening I heard my parents talking in their bedroom. They sounded quite concerned. It seemed that someone else from our parish had left the convent, ran up lots of debt, and then had psychiatric problems. Her parents were left with the bills.

"Will Mary be okay? She doesn't even have a job," I heard my mom ask.

I could understand their concern; I was worried, too.

The next day, Dad and I went to a Dodge dealer to order a new car. Dad had purchased cars there before and knew the manager.

"This is my daughter, Mary. She used to be a nun," Dad said, when he introduced me.

He ordered the cheapest car they had with nothing but a simple radio in it, not even air conditioning. My dad then co-signed for my brand new Dodge Dart. The debt was covered fully by payments, which I would make over four years.

"It will take some time to prep the car," the manager said, "We'll do it this afternoon and you can pick it up tomorrow."

"No, she needs it today," Dad said. "I'm headed for an appointment. Mary can wait and drive it home."

While I waited for the car, I roamed around the showroom looking at the other vehicles. An older, gray-haired man who was not connected with the dealership, approached me at the water cooler and said, "You shouldn't be driving an inexpensive car; you should have a sporty car. My friends and I could set you up in a penthouse, give you a convertible and all you would have to do is entertain us and our friends on the weekend. How about it?"

If only he knew that I had just come home from the convent four days before! His proposal was so ridiculous that I burst into laughter, turned and walked away across the showroom. My car was soon ready and I drove it home.

When I left the convent, the Reverend Mother of the Sisters of St. Joseph had indicated that if I had trouble getting a job, they would hire me, but for obvious reasons, they would rather not. I was determined to get a job on my own, so early the following morning, I went for a job interview at St. Clement's Catholic School, which was run by Dominican nuns.

From my resume, the principal, Sister Mary Jude, knew that I had been a nun with the Sisters of St. Joseph. They needed a teacher for the second grade and she offered the position to me. I felt that would not be as demanding on me as teaching the upper grades, so I accepted, asking Sister Mary Jude not to tell anyone that I had been a nun. I still had not completed college, so she sent for a teaching certificate for me.

I was excited that my new life was falling into place. The new school year was scheduled to start in three weeks, and I had no doubt that I would be able to handle my debts. My parents were ecstatic!

I spent several weeks preparing my classroom, looking over the texts and preparing lesson plans, attending daily Mass at St. Rita's, our neighborhood church, and now I would be able to see my sister, Gracie.

I had been calling Gracie ever since I came home, but now, I had time to visit with her, baby-sit my nephews and occasionally stay overnight. That was exciting. We talked for a long time into the night. Gracie offered tips on makeup and gave me some ideas on hairstyles. I was grateful for all the help she gave me.

One day, Gracie received a phone call from a neighbor asking, "What's wrong? Why aren't you friendly anymore? You didn't even wave at me."

When I was out in the yard, the neighbor had waved at me, thinking I was Gracie, and I didn't pay any attention to her!

"My twin sister is visiting," Gracie told her, laughing. "I'll tell her that in the future, she should look and wave at everybody."

We might no longer be identical, but from a distance who would know?

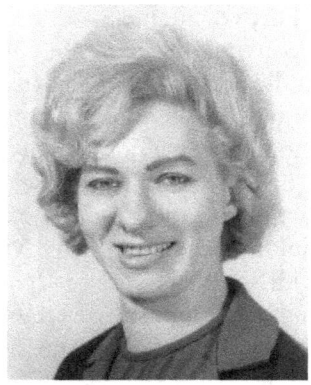

1964. Just out of the convent! Notice the hang lip, wider nose, jutting jaw, higher cheekbones, coarse and oily skin. I was 30 years old and weighed 103 pounds.

Within the first two weeks of classes, two of the nuns came into my classroom to chat. Their request took me by surprise.

"We've been watching you," one of them said. "You have such lovely clothes. They're so stylish with light, bright colors. You just seem to 'have it all together.'"

"There's a teacher here who left the convent several years ago," the other said, "and we were wondering if you could help her. She always wears darker clothing with no style. She dresses as though she is still a nun." The sister paused. "She really needs help. Would you talk to her?"

If these nuns only knew I had left the convent myself less than a month previously.

My clothes were all new; so, of course, they looked great; but inwardly, I was quite pleased at the complement.

The sisters gave me the other teacher's name, Joan Higgins, and I stopped by her classroom to introduce myself. I was going to a fashion show the following week, and I invited her along. At the show, I encouraged her to buy a brightly colored suit that looked lovely with her dark hair.

We became friends and, after the show, I told Joan that I had been a nun. She didn't act surprised. Some years later, still my good friend, she told me that when we met, she knew immediately that I had been a nun. My long hair surprised her, but the indentation in my forehead caused by wearing the habit was quite obvious. It had taken several months for that mark to disappear. The Dominicans hadn't noticed because their habits were made differently and didn't make the tell-tale mark on the forehead.

My first paycheck arrived, and I immediately gave some money to my parents. I knew it would take them completely by surprise.

"I will pay you the same amount for room and board twice a month," I told them.

41

Later that night, I could hear the excitement in their voices, "She's going to be just fine," I heard my dad say.

They were relieved, and so was I.

Teaching is such a rewarding experience and also lots of fun. No two days are ever the same. Sometimes, children will say that they can't do a particular assignment.

"American ends in I can!" I told them.

Often, students responded with groans, but they learned.

Self-worth is so important to every youngster. I constantly reminded parents at parent-teacher functions that if they helped their children develop good self-images and self-worth, they would be giving them something worth more than money.

"Never let anyone put a label on your child," I told the parents. "Name calling can do irreparable harm. Don't put labels on yourselves, either," I continued. "Labels set limits and can cripple."

I enjoyed teaching, and I loved the children and determined that teaching would be my mission in life. I attended daily Mass with the students before classes began in the mornings.

The dating scenario did not enter my mind, and I never considered pursuing it; however, associate teachers and friends, well, that was a different story. They began to suggest that I meet this person or that person, so eventually, I allowed myself to consider the possibility that perhaps I might someday meet someone who was right for me. Marriage just might be in God's plan for me. Still, I would allow God's Spirit to lead me.

Joan and I became good friends and often went out to lunch together. We decided to go to a nearby bar to have a few drinks. Maybe, we would meet some nice men. We soon found that the men we met there were not the type of guys we were looking for. I met one man named Bill, who seemed okay, but I didn't encourage him. We had a drink and I said, "Thanks" and "Good-bye."

If teaching were going to be my life's work, I needed to obtain my college degree. With that in mind, I signed up for an evening class at Wayne State University in January of 1965. I found that many of the classes I had taken at Nazareth College were not acceptable at Wayne State. I would almost be starting over, but it definitely was something I had to pursue.

I was still plagued with headaches, but they were not as severe as they had been in the fifties. I still weighed in at one-hundred-three pounds and I continued to have problems with fatigue, dizziness deep within my head, and extreme sensitivity to light.

These symptoms made driving to the university a couple of nights each week a problem. Taking on the additional work also caused the exhaustion I still experienced to become worse. Teaching all day, driving to Wayne State and committing time to my studies was just not working out. I tried to stay committed to my classes, but after about five weeks, I had to quit.

The exhaustion stayed with me, even after dropping my course. In an attempt to resolve the problem, I began to retire early and get lots of rest on the weekends. I slept-in till noon on Saturdays with no bell to wake me up and on Sunday, I slept-in and attended the twelve o'clock Mass to worship my God.

In spite of the continuing physical difficulties, my life seemed to be progressing smoothly. I didn't know that it was about to take a sharp turn.

Chapter 7

Enter Bob

Late one Friday afternoon in February of 1965, the phone rang. It was for me.

"My name is Bob," a masculine voice on the line said. "You don't know me, and I don't know you, but there's a fellow who works for me who you also don't know, but he knows your brother-in-law, who said you were in town, and how about a date? Your brother-in-law got the okay from your sister and gave me your phone number."

Bob was so nervous about calling me that one phrase ran into another in a confused rush. It must have taken a lot of courage for him to call me, so I said yes. No one had told him that I used to be a nun and I didn't either.

Bob arrived at my house the next evening and when my mother met him, she hurried into my bedroom.

"He really looks like a nice guy!" Mom said.

On that snowy evening, Bob took me to a classy restaurant at Pine Knob, a nearby ski resort. It was a romantic, dimly-lit setting with a gentleman playing classical music at the piano, a full wall of windows looking out at the skiers, who were coasting down the hillside with flashlights in the dark, creating a beautiful view.

Bob told me that he was an engineer at the Chrysler Corporation. He said he lived in a home that he owned.

Ummm, I began to be suspicious. *Here is a man in his thirties, driving a four-door sedan, and owing a home. Could he be married?*

When I questioned him, he assured me that he was not, nor ever had been married. His father died when he was a baby, and his mother had never remarried, he explained. Bob had purchased the house for his mother. It belonged to him and he had lived in it, since her death the previous year. It was a small house, but sufficient for his needs.

The evening ended at The Top of the Flame, a fantastic Far Eastern bar overlooking downtown Detroit and the river front. I couldn't have imagined a better first date.

Bob continued to wine and dine me. We went to the Fisher Theater to see Dolly Parton and Frank Sinatra and to Broadway shows. He took me to a night club across the border in Windsor, Canada to see Jimmy Durante and Wayne Newton. To make it easier on the pocketbook, we also went to movies and other events.

Before we were engaged, I turned his invitations down from time to time. He seemed like such a wonderful person, so easy to talk with and I knew I was falling in love, but I didn't want things to happen too fast. Later, I found that he had taken someone else to see Harry Belafonte and other events. When I asked him about it, he said that he had purchased the tickets before he asked me. I had to admit that he couldn't waste such expensive tickets.

Classes ended in the middle of June. In July, I went with my parents to visit my ninety-five-year-old grandpa in Missouri.

I welcomed time away from Bob. I knew I was in love with him and believed that he loved me, too. I felt that he might be on the verge of asking me to marry him and I wanted time to pray about such a serious decision.

Upon my return from Missouri in August 1965, the phone rang one morning at seven a.m. It was Bob. It was urgent; he had to see me right away, he said. He had to make a quick stop at his office and then he would pick me up.

Soon, his car pulled up in our driveway. He helped me into the front seat and drove to a nearby park. I was almost shaking, I was so nervous. *Why the urgency? Was he going to propose at last?*

We got out of the car at the park and Bob walked with me over to a nearby bench and began to kiss me, over and over. He asked me to sit down and he knelt on one knee and asked, "Will you marry me?"

"Yes!"

I felt relief and happiness all rolled into one. It was such an exciting morning. We continued to talk and kiss on the park bench. Suddenly, Bob realized that he had better get back to work.

"Before you go," I said. "I have something to tell you."

Then, I nervously told him that I had been a nun.

"So what?" he answered. "I love you, Mary. The guys at the office complained that I've been bumping into doors and not paying attention to what's going on. They said that they can't take it anymore, and I should go out and propose to you."

I'd gotten lipstick on his collar, so he had to stop at his house for a clean shirt, before dropping me off at home. On the drive from the park, Bob had asked me if I wanted a new house or would I prefer to move into his house and spend the money on an extensive European honeymoon. I hadn't seen his house, but I chose Europe.

When we got to his house, he realized that he had left the house key at the office, but he quickly broke in.

While Bob changed into a clean shirt, I looked around the little house located on a quiet street in northern Detroit. I thought it was cute with its two bedrooms and a one-and-a-half detached garage. *Yes, it will be fun living here*, I thought, *and I'm going to have a European honeymoon!*

Later, we discussed the fact that I would be thirty-two by the end of our honeymoon and we had agreed that if we were to have children, we should let nature take its course. If I should get pregnant right away, so be it. We both thought that four children would make a nice family.

We planned the wedding for April 16, 1966, almost seven months away. My sister, Patty, was pregnant and due in October of 1965. She would be in my wedding party and my twin sister, Gracie, would be my matron of honor. How much more wonderful could my life be?

I had prayed often for God's blessings on my life and now, one of His many blessings came in the persona of this wonderful man named "Bob."

In the fall of 1965, I still taught at St. Clement's school, but I had changed to the seventh grade. I was excited about teaching Junior High and was prepared for all the responsibilities that go with it.

In early December, I noticed a vaginal discharge of blood. I had never had my own doctor, so I was happy when my dad said he would take me to meet Dr. Pellman, my parent's family doctor. My dad introduced me to his doctor the same way he had been introducing me to all of his friends, "This is my daughter, who was a nun." I had gritted my teeth and smiled every time it happened; but, finally, after this time, I asked if I could just be his daughter—and leave off the nun part!

Dr. Pellman did a vaginal check-up and said, "Your dad said you are engaged to be married. Are you pregnant?"

"Positively, no!" I responded.

Dr. Pellman asked me a few more questions, which indicated that he thought I must be naïve.

"How far do you let your fiancé touch you? Does he just touch your back, or does he go farther?"

"Absolutely, I am not pregnant!"

He said that he would have to perform a dilation and curettage, more commonly known as a D & C, but also known more flippantly as a "dusting and cleaning." I would enter the hospital during the Christmas vacation.

"I will schedule you for December 27th," he said. "You will be in the hospital for three days."

Dr. Pellman's nurse made the arrangements and had me enter the hospital through the emergency entrance. After the surgery, Dr. Pellman greeted me in the recovery room with good news.

"I removed large polyps at the mouth of the uterus, but everything else looked good and I didn't have to perform a D & C," he said. "You'll be moved into a room as soon as one is available."

I had been warned that at this time of year, hospitals are often filled to capacity; therefore, when I was later rolled into a private room, I was relieved.

The relief was short-lived. Within a few minutes, a woman came into the room and asked, "What did you have?"

Before I could answer, a young girl came by and asked the same question. When I told them that I had polyps removed, they both responded, "Oh, yeah!"

Just then, a nurse came in and ordered them out of the room.

"She's not one of you," she said, "so move out of here."

"Where am I?" I asked.

"You're on the unwed mother's floor."

What a surprise!

After dinner, I saw attendants roll a woman on a stretcher into the next room. Later, I heard her calling the nurse for pain medication.

A nurse called in to her, "You got yourself into this mess, if you want pain medication, walk down to the nursing station and pick it up yourself."

I was angry. The nurses were paid to do their jobs and had no right to condemn these women or treat them so roughly. The nurses responded to my needs very quickly and brought my pain medication when I needed it.

A fourteen-year-old girl came into my room later.

"This is my second baby. My mom rents out my bedroom at night for money and there is nothing I can do about it," she told me.

Meanwhile, the nurses continued to tell patients to pick up their own meds. By 11 p.m., I called for the nurse who supervised the night shift. On the phone, I told her what was happening to these women and how the nursing staff should be helping, not hurting, their patients.

Apparently, my remarks had caused quite a stir. Dr. Pellman came into my room early the next morning.

"We have to get you out of here," he said. "I heard what you did and some of the nurses are very angry with you."

He signed me out and my dad picked me up and took me home to recuperate and to prepare for my wedding.

Chapter 8

European Honeymoon

Many of my students were involved in the wedding, when Bob and I were married. Some of them made pompoms for decorating the cars, while others made table decorations or small gifts for us. Several of the parents commented that they were happy to have their children see such a great success story. So many young people were getting married right out of high school. The parents were pleased that their children were exposed to a role model in a teacher who had pursued an education, had a career, and now, a storybook wedding and honeymoon. Of course, they never knew I had been a nun.

I had given my notice to quit teaching. Bob and I just assumed that I would become pregnant soon and that my time would be taken up with our own children. The parents were told that the substitute teacher would follow my teaching plans for the remainder of the year and would be the full-time teacher for that grade during the next school year. They were relieved to know that their children's education would have continuity.

The wedding rehearsal and dinner were on Thursday night. Friday evening, April 15th, Bob and I dined at an Italian restaurant and then planned to drive out to the airport to pick up Bob's relatives coming in from Pennsylvania. Beaming at each other, excited about the wedding the next day, when my dinner arrived, I bit into a piece of shrimp and one of my front teeth broke off at the gum line. It had been capped independently from the other front teeth.

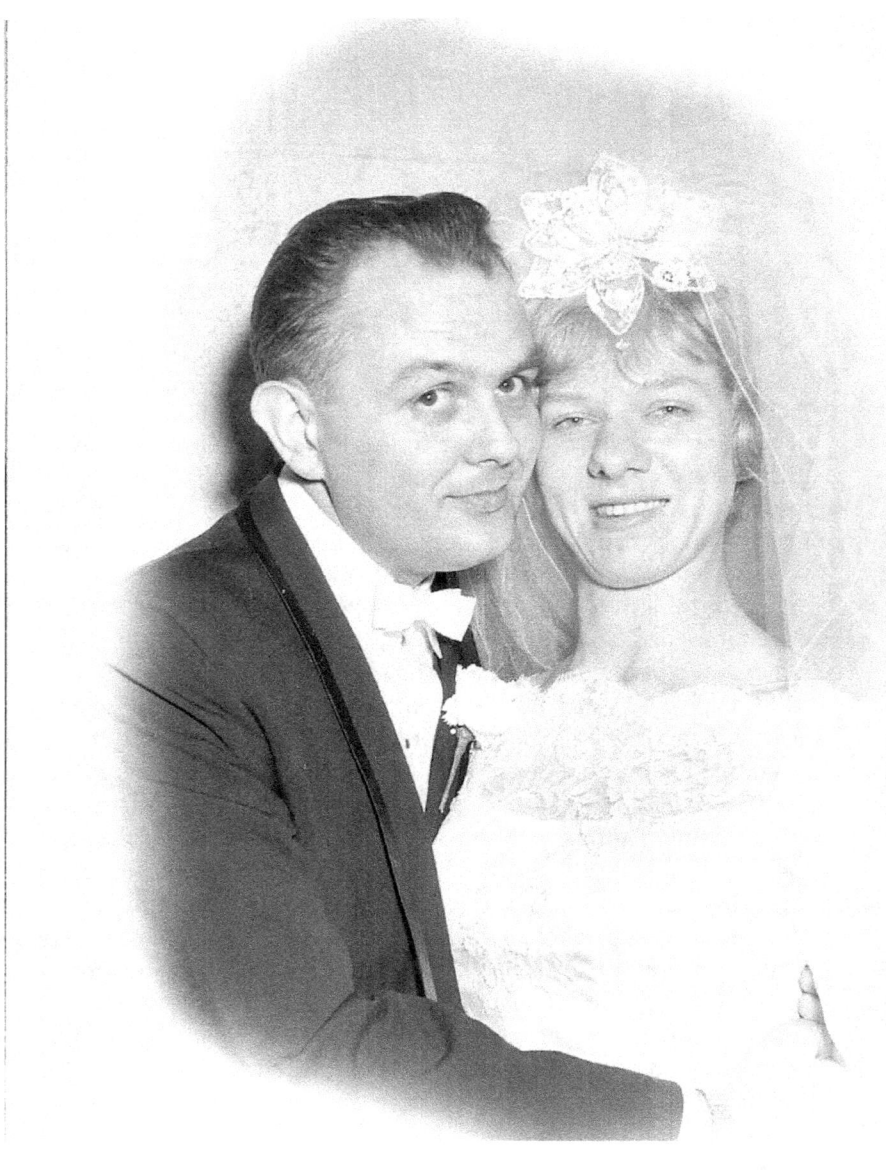

Our wedding picture—April 16, 1966. Compare my facial features with the picture on page 85. See how much facial growth occurred between 1966 and 1969, caused by an actively growing pituitary tumor.

"Bob," I cried, "No way can I get married tomorrow with my front tooth missing and our honeymoon! I can't go on a long trip with a broken tooth."

I was completely distraught.

Bob quickly called his Uncle Ken to pick up the relatives from Pennsylvania. We left our dinners and drove to Bob's house. I didn't have a dentist. Bob called his dentist and I was in the dental chair that night having a peg tooth put into my mouth. Bob had saved the day! He invited the dentist and his wife to our wedding the next day and they did attend.

Late on a Saturday morning in mid-April, many of the nuns, teachers and students witnessed our wedding at St. Rita's Catholic Church. I was thrilled to have them share this great joyous occasion with me, along with my wonderful family. My sisters looked beautiful in their gowns and the wedding ceremony was more than beautiful, as I became Mrs. Robert J. Stevens, and Bob and I vowed to belong to each other for better or worse, in sickness and in health, till death do we part. The celebration lasted far into the night.

The afternoon after the wedding, Bob said he wanted to measure my waistline. His relatives had commented about how slim I appeared and he wanted to know *how* slim. I weighed about 105 pounds and his tape measure showed that my waist was 22 inches, bust 34, and hips 34. A good size for a bride, he declared.

On Monday, April 18 we flew to New York City, where I had my passport changed from Mary J. McFadden to Mary J. Stevens; then, we flew on to Spain to begin our honeymoon in Europe. My menstrual period, no longer precise, had been late the month before, and it started on April 18 at Metropolitan airport, just before we left for Spain. What great timing!

Bob had made special arrangements—a travel agent picked us up at each airport in an unmarked car, handled our

luggage, and coordinated any reservation changes or deviations from
our plans. He had planned it well! Together, we selected the locations, excursions, and sites we wanted to see.

We first arrived in beautiful Spain for the yearly festival in Seville. Outstanding! Cobblestone streets, gorgeous archaic buildings, orange trees and palm trees—it seemed so unreal. Dressed in their native costumes, the people danced in the streets just as in the movies. Palaces, bull fights, art museums, fabulous churches, mountain ranges—a honeymoon I would never forget. Then we traveled on to the palaces of Madrid and neighboring sites. We dined in restaurants that I later saw shown on television travel shows. What fabulous experiences.

Paris in the springtime! The most romantic spot on earth. It was early May and all of Paris was in bloom. We dined at a restaurant down the boulevard from our hotel, and when we went on a nightclub tour that evening, the guide pointed out the same restaurant and said, "That is the most expensive restaurant on the Champs-Elysees."

"I know," Bob responded. "My wife and I just dined there. The food was fantastic, but my wife's menu had no prices. You know what that means!"

During the day after touring the historical sites, including Notre Dame, the Arc-de-Triumphe, Montmartre district, where the streets are filled with artists selling their paintings, the Louvre, and the Eiffel tower, we enjoyed dinner on the Bateau Mouche—a boat ride on the River Seine.

Our journey took us to Nice, where we were driven into the French Alps and dined at a mountain top restaurant called the Chez D'or. The Chez D'or offered a vast view of the Mediterranean Sea, Monte Carlo, and an American Navy ship, a destroyer, docked out in the bay.

We gambled in the Casino at Monte Carlo, where there is a strict dress code and swam in the warm waters of the Mediterranean. In the ancient city of Rome, we toured the Vatican, and stood amid the ruins of the Coliseum. It was moving to see that huge amphitheater where Christians were thrown to the lions in the first and second century.

Later in Venice, I felt nausea in the morning. Bob wondered if it could be seasickness from the gondolas and motorboats, but I was accustomed to boats. No, I began to think I must be pregnant.

The daily nausea was over by noon, and so we adjusted to sleeping till noon, sightseeing in the afternoon and enjoying the nightlife. Bob knew that I did not have a lot of stamina and often needed extra rest; however, another change occurred. My breast size started to balloon. Huge. Bob could not believe what was happening to me. Neither could I. We made a quick trip to the store for new bras.

In romantic Venice, we visited San Marco's Square beside St. Mark's Cathedral and motor boated out to the Island of Murano, famed for its blown glass. In the evenings, we rode gondolas through the canals.

When the rigollatta of gondoliers is celebrated, people in gondoliers float through the canals, while in larger boats, entertainers strum guitars and sing beautiful Italian songs, as they slowly wind under the Bridge of Sighs, named after the prisoners, who sighed walking over it on their way to prison or their executions. Finally, the boats drift out into the Grand Canal leading to open water.

One night, I stepped into the gondola and Bob stepped back to allow another woman to come aboard. She and her husband were Americans and were excited to meet us. She chose to sit by me and all Bob could do was groan as he conversed with her husband. The normally polite Bob told me that his stepping aside was over. That night we enjoyed a romantic gondola ride sitting side by side.

Before it ended, our trip took us to the Alps, Munich, Bavaria and then to Vienna, where we visited palaces in the Vienna Woods. It was a fantastic honeymoon.

Unfortunately, in addition to my swollen breasts, other physical changes had been occurring. I had bought leather gloves in Spain, and by the time we went through the Alps and on to Bavaria, my hands had gotten so much larger that they no longer fit. My shoe size went from a nine quad (very slim) to a D width. I justified the changes by saying they probably happened because I was pregnant. I never thought they might be caused by anything else.

Coming home, we had a lengthy flight across the Atlantic Ocean going from Vienna to New York. The plane encountered numerous storms, had to rise higher to avoid some, and had to go off course to circumvent others. It was a rough ride. As we were getting closer to our destination, several passengers, who traveled that flight frequently, commented that the plane had changed its course, this time for no apparent reason.

The pilot's voice came over the speaker system.

"We are low on fuel. We cannot make it to Kennedy Airport. We will try to land in Boston."

"What do they mean by 'try'?" I asked Bob.

People on the plane were visibly upset. Some were clutching their children. Bob and I looked at each other.

"We had a great honeymoon. Is this going to be the end for us? All we can do is to pray and trust in God," we agreed.

The pilot's voice came across again.

"We cannot land in Boston because of heavy fog, and we cannot make it to Kennedy Airport."

The stewardesses began passing out free liquor to everyone, as many drinks as you wanted.

"We must land in Boston," the pilot finally announced, "They have had heavy fog conditions for days. We will be landing at the far end of the airport."

I thought, *That's a good idea. We certainly don't want to smash into the terminal.*

We passengers were advised to secure any loose pieces of luggage and to get into crash position with pillows over our heads. I sat up to see the action. It was early evening but the cloud cover and fog, made it quite dark.

Fire engines and ambulances with lights flashing raced down on either side of the runway, as we descended into the foggy airport. Perhaps their lights helped the pilot to see his way. Finally, the wheels touched down. The plane bounced down the runway, but amid loud cheers and happy faces, everyone was relieved to feel land beneath the plane.

After being transported by buses from the plane to the terminal, we found people milling around. Planes had been stuck on the ground in the fog, on and off for several days. It was predicted that it would soon clear, and we heard an announcement that a plane would leave for Detroit Metropolitan Airport later that night. I was so tired, so exhausted. How Bob got us on that one plane, I will never know, but we were on it and arrived safely in Detroit.

"You must be God's fair-haired child." Bob commented that night. "He does protect you. Whenever something goes wrong, I want to make sure that I am with you."

I hoped Bob was right. It was a protection I would certainly need in the coming year.

Chapter 9

Lisa Joins Us

Bob and I, together with our new identities as Mr. and Mrs. Robert J. Stevens, returned from our honeymoon in time for the last week of school. I had promised my students that I would be back for that week to say goodbye to them. I kept my promise. The students asked so many questions about our European trip that I shared pictures with them of some of the exciting places we visited.

The principal, Sister Mary Jude, requested that I consider coming back just to teach art classes to the Junior High students, but I couldn't. I was pregnant!

"My next career will be motherhood," I told her.

Bob and I estimated that I had become pregnant in Paris, as my symptoms began to show up when we reached Venice at the end of May. We were both so excited to have a baby on the way.

I called my twin sister, Gracie, to share our happiness with her and to ask the name of her ob/gyn. It was a Doctor Juno, Gracie told me and I made an appointment for early July. I never kept the appointment, because in late June, I began to experience problems and had a miscarriage.

Bob and I were both emotional over this loss, and my mom consoled us by saying, "You got pregnant once, so it will probably happen again." That didn't lessen the sting of the baby we had lost, but it gave us something to look forward to.

With no reason to stay at home now, I decided to sign up for a teaching position in the fall.

"If you need a reason to stay home," Bob said, "let's get a dog."

We bought "Buddy," a black Labrador puppy, but a dog

wasn't a good reason to stay home. I began negotiating for a teaching position at a public school. The position would have put me in charge of team teaching for a junior high school. I was surprised and a little intimidated, because of the four teachers, I was the only one without a degree and I would be the team leader.

A curve ball came at me again during the summer of 1966, when I again became pregnant. Bob and I were so happy, until in the early stages, signs of another miscarriage began to occur. Fearful that I might lose the baby, my obstetrician prescribed medication and ordered me to stay on complete bed rest. That effectively ended my negotiation for the teaching position.

I continually prayed, *God, bless us in our marriage, but especially bless us with this baby.*

Bob and I were both excited with this new pregnancy. We immediately started discussing baby names and began planning the decorations for the nursery. By the third or fourth month, my pregnancy seemed secure. I resumed some normal activities; however, I was once again continually plagued with exhaustion. Would I make my due date at the end of April?

During this time, Bob and I took a class on "Baby Care." The instructor taught us how to care for a baby's health, as well as feeding, changing diapers and bathing, all much needed information for both of us.

I went for my annual checkup with my optometrist, who had prescribed contact lenses the year before. I was happy with the contacts, but apparently, the optometrist noted a problem. My optic nerves were blue, which usually is a sign of pressure on them. The doctor noted what he had seen on my chart, but never mentioned it to me, deciding to wait a year to determine whether there might be other changes. If I had known, I would have gone to an ophthalmologist for a better diagnosis, but that didn't happen.

Throughout this pregnancy, I spent much of my time resting. I felt so tired; I could easily have slept around the clock on many days. One day toward the end of April, false labor sent me running to the hospital, followed by several repeat performances. Dr. Juno recommended that I come into the hospital and let him induce labor. We agreed, but after three failed attempts, the doctor left for his vacation. We knew that we were in the capable hands of his associate, but felt enormously frustrated.

Our emotions were running over. Even Bob's fellow workers offered him advice.

"Drive Mary over bumpy roads."

"Pray for stormy weather. That's when babies usually arrive."

Dr. Juno's associate offered different advice.

"We don't see where you should have any problem with this delivery; perhaps, we were off on the due date. That happens. Your early symptoms may have been due to something else. The baby will come when it's ready."

Unfortunately, that statement turned out not to be true. Again, I had labor pains and Bob drove me to the hospital around noon on June 9, 1967. Near midnight, after long hours of labor, Dr. Juno, having returned from his vacation, preformed an emergency caesarean section.

Lisa, our beautiful baby girl, arrived with blue eyes and blondish fuzz on her nearly bald head; she weighed in at eight pounds and resembled me. Immediately after her birth, the nurse showed her to me, but I was so groggy from medications that all I noticed were her big feet. I was so relieved just to see her, that I prayed over and over again in thanksgiving to my God.

Bob left the hospital around midnight and returned about 7 a.m. with a pink football. During my pregnancy, he had purchased a football in case we had a son. Now that he had a daughter, he had gone home and painted it pink during the night. Lisa still has her pink football.

When Bob returned to his office at Chrysler, the members of the entire department stood up and applauded, happy that his duress—and by extension, theirs!—was over and he finally had his baby daughter.

When the wheels of the bassinet carrying my baby rolled quietly into my room for her first feeding, I was excited but still too exhausted to hold her. My huge breasts, filled with milk, hurt, and disappointment overwhelmed me. I wanted so much to nurse my baby, but I just couldn't. Surely, this was more than normal exhaustion after giving birth, but the doctor had not suggested that there might be a problem with my health.

The nurse's aide gave Lisa a bottle and placed her into bed beside me. She lay there quietly as I touched her and talked to her. She was so beautiful. I couldn't believe I finally had a baby.

When the next feeding time arrived, and the nurse brought Lisa back for her bottle, she again lay very quietly. Soon, the nurse took her to the nursery for the night.

Tired, I went right to sleep, as usual, but woke suddenly in the middle of the night, terrified!

"Something is wrong with my baby. My baby is mute," I screamed.

I called for the nurse to bring Lisa into my room.

"I know something is wrong with my baby. She can't cry."

The nurse brought Lisa into the room, smacked her on the bottom, and she cried. What a relief. My baby was normal. My terror was unfounded.

Thank you, God!

My exhaustion continued to be so extreme that upon leaving the hospital, Dr. Juno insisted that I must have someone to assist me at home in caring for the baby. He said I could not take care of her by myself. Bob said that he would take a vacation from work and, of course, my mother said she would help.

The first night at home was so exciting. Bob said that he would get up when Lisa cried and he would give her a bottle, so that I could sleep. Morning came with no sound from our baby.

"What time during the night did you give Lisa a bottle?" I asked Bob.

"I never woke up," he said.

Here it was morning and no sound from a hungry, new-born baby.

Oh, my God. She's probably dead.

We both raced into Lisa's room to find a happy baby, who, apparently, had slept through the night. From that day forward, she slept through every night, unless she was teething.

Bob took his vacation from work and gave Lisa her first bath, with my mother watching nearby. For weeks, my mother and Bob took care of both the baby and me; while I gradually progressed until the day came that I finally took over her total care. *What a wonderful experience! Thank you, God.*

Just prior to our marriage, I had chosen a European honeymoon over having a new house. Now, with the prospect of a growing family, I realized that I'd really like to have that new house. Bob agreed and Lisa, Bob and I had a great deal of fun house hunting. At last, we found a builder's model that would be perfect for us provided the builder make some changes in the design.

We had him add a large walk-in closet and a full bathroom attached to the master bedroom, enlarge the family room, add a twenty-foot first floor laundry room, and coaxed him into letting Bob design the fireplace for the family room. Now Lisa, Bob and I made frequent trips out to the building site, watching our new ranch home being custom built from the basement up.

Meanwhile, I went to a neighborhood Tupperware party and announced that we were moving. A lady at the party immediately commented, "I want to buy your house."

So within a few weeks, the price was negotiated and we sold our little two bedroom house in Detroit.

Chapter 10

You're Not Identical

January 1968 arrived, and with it moving day. Bob, Lisa, Buddy, our black Labrador retriever, and I moved into our new house, a brick ranch in the suburbs of Detroit. Meanwhile, for almost nine months after Lisa's birth I experienced severe lactation (heavy milk seepage from the breast), no menstrual periods, severe nausea in the form of morning sickness—all the signs that I might be pregnant again, but pregnancy tests were negative.

Dry mouth and increased urination, suggested diabetes, but those tests also produced negative results. I made weekly, then monthly visits to my ob/gyn, Dr. Juno, for checkups and testing.

"I know Mary's twin sister," Dr. Juno said on one visit, in a side comment to his receptionist. "She's one of my patients, too, but they certainly aren't identical."

"We were identical," I quickly responded, feeling I had to set the record straight. "We used to lead processions and parades. I can bring in pictures to prove it."

At the doctor's request, I brought the pictures in the next day and upon viewing them, he suddenly realized what my health problem might really be.

"I've studied and read about acromegaly, but I have never seen a case of it. Acromegaly is a pituitary disorder. I think that might be your problem."

"Where is the pituitary located?" I asked.

"At the base of the brain," he answered.

I thought that meant the pituitary would be located at the back of the head, just above the neck: *an easy place for the doctor to operate, if that proved to be my problem.* My gynecologist scheduled me to meet with a specialist in the neurology department of a nearby hospital that same month.

Finally, a diagnosis! Acromegaly, caused by a pituitary tumor and discovered completely by accident! Being a twin saved my life. If the doctor hadn't made that passing comment, it may never have been found. Praise God. Had I stayed in the convent, an accidental discovery probably would never have taken place. Thank you. Thank you God.

During past years, when friends and relatives saw my sister, Gracie, and me together, they accepted my different physical appearance as being natural, probably thinking that twins, even identical twins, change physically as they get older, Now we know that is not true.

I met with the neurologist.

"Acromegaly," he told me, "is usually caused by a tumor, usually benign, located in the pituitary gland. Apparently a cell in the pituitary gland begins to grow abnormally, probably activated by something in the person's life—puberty, birth of a child, change of life, or something else that stimulated that cell to begin to grow. The type of growth problems the person experiences depends on the direction of the growth of the tumor."

In my case, it was probably activated at puberty, and its growth started to become evident at about the age of seventeen.

The neurologist further stated, "The pituitary gland controls practically everything in your body, and can effect your hormones, your glands; even your heart. That is why your birthing muscles didn't work. *Well, at least that mystery is solved.*

The thought of having a brain tumor really scared me. Knowing that a tumor might have been growing inside my head, causing all these health problems and physical changes over the years was devastating. I prayed. I worried. Then I prayed some more.

Whenever I drove, I became aware that I was losing my peripheral vision. I had to quickly turn my head back and forth to see oncoming traffic from the sides; but I was in denial that I had a vision problem. I didn't want to stop driving.

The neurologists determined that I should be admitted to the hospital for extensive testing. From the numerous physical changes I exhibited, the doctors indicated I had acromegaly, the result of quite a large tumor. Brain surgery was inevitable.

"The pituitary is located behind the eyes, in the middle of the head in a bony structure called the sella turcica," one neurologist explained to me.

He showed me a diagram to clarify the location. Now I knew it was not in the back of the head, just above the neck, but in the middle of my head. Big difference! By this time, I was really scared.

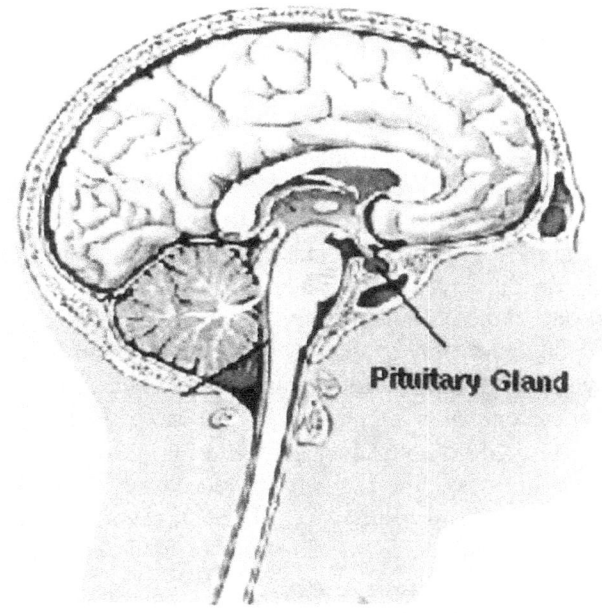

Picture compliments of the PNA Network—Pituitary Patient Resource Guide—Volume VI, Number 4, August 1998 issue.

While driving home, I prayed out loud. God has always been an integral part of my life. I begged Him to come to my aid. *God, please send Your Holy Spirit to touch me and heal me, lift my spirit and keep me calm.*

My mother was baby sitting with Lisa and when I picked her up that day, I shared what I had learned with my mother.

"I may have to enter the hospital for testing for a brain tumor," I said. "I am really scared."

My mother put her arms around me, hugged me and tried to console me.

"If I have to go in the hospital, will you take care of Lisa?"

"Of course Dad and I will take care of her," she said, hugging me tightly.

At the dinner table that night, I told Bob the bad news. We had surmised that I would have to eventually have tests at the hospital, but now reality hit us. We sat quietly at the table lost in our own thoughts and staring blankly into space. Lisa, sitting in her high chair, sensed something was wrong. She kept looking from one of us to the other, and finally she burst into tears.

The poor baby. Of course she didn't understand, but she knew something was wrong from the strength of the tension in the room. Together, we reached out to her, hugged her, and played with her. Together we decided to control our emotions and wait for the test results. We had Lisa to consider, and had to be optimistic for ourselves and for her.

Several days later, the neurology department notified me of the doctors' decision that extensive testing would probably be followed by surgery, and it would have to be done immediately. The tumor could cause an aneurysm or, because of its size, even affect the brain. I could go insane, they said.

Visions of the psychiatric ward I had visited with Sister Mary Benedict filled my mind. I heard Dr. X's voice shouting, "You need a psychiatrist." *Stop! You have to be calm. You have to be positive.*

Mom and Dad renewed their agreement to care for Lisa. We took her to my parents' home on Monday, May 6, and settled her into their house, crib and all. Then Bob and I went out to dinner and a movie to try to relax. Of course, I was still worried and scared. Fortunately, Bob hid his concern much better than I did.

I was admitted to the hospital on my birthday, Tuesday, May 7, 1968 (Happy thirty-fourth birthday to me) to undergo a barrage of tests, torture tests. Having determined that I was hypoglycemic, a variety of tests had been scheduled to be performed over the next couple of weeks.

First came an angiogram, a diagnostic procedure in which a technician inserted a catheter into an artery near my shoulder then threaded it upward toward my brain to search for any blockage in my arteries. Technicians injected dye through the catheter and took x-rays to give the doctor a picture of the blood vessels feeding my head, brain stem and neck.

I experienced extreme pain during the more than two hours that it took to complete this procedure. The dye felt like fire continuously shooting through my arteries. I imagined that electrocution must be very much like this test. The technician constantly reminded me not to move or the x-rays would have to be taken over and more dye inserted. I cooperated fully. I wanted the procedure to be finished quickly, but it took hours. Test results indicated that there was no blockage in my arteries.

Vision testing confirmed that my peripheral vision had been affected and that my visual field had been limited (tunnel vision). An additional result of the initial testing showed that I had an enlarged thyroid with a goiter. Most goiters appear as growths on the neck. Mine grew inward into my throat.

An electroencephalogram (EEG), a test that measures and records the electrical activity of the brain, came next. One of the nurses warned me that when I finished with the EEG I would need to wash my hair. I soon found out why. She put a goopy substance in many locations on my scalp where she placed electrodes in order to do the recording and graphing.

The reality of the procedure surprised me. In order to get a more accurate reading, they put the pins directly into my scalp. Again I received a stern warning. "Don't move or the electrodes will pop out and have to be reinserted." Finally, each one was pressed firmly into my scalp, as I bit my lips to keep from crying out, and the reading and graphing was quickly completely.

At that time, there were no magnetic resonance imaging (MRI) or computerized axial tomography (CAT) scans available in that hospital, so my last test was a pneumoencephalogram, requiring the insertion of enough air into the spine to move the air mass up to the brain area. Then by mechanically twirling and rotating the chair, the air mass moved to various parts of my brain while x-rays were taken. During this procedure, I was securely locked into the rotating chair.

"Just pretend you are in outer space and there is no gravity as we turn you around and upside down," the technicians and doctors repeatedly told me and continually reminded me not to move during the x-rays or it would take that much longer. As it was, it took hours, unbelievable, endless hours.

I screamed repeatedly! The pain and nausea were excruciating, and I couldn't have any anesthetic during this ordeal. It had to be accurate. One of the neurologists indicated to me that this test could kill a patient. With all the pain I endured, I believed it then and I believe it now. I had been required to sign an authorization prior to the test to accept that risk.

This final test had been necessary for my doctors   to determine the size and exact location of the pituitary tumor, and the approach required for the surgery. After the test I had to lie flat for twenty-four hours to avoid getting what they characterized as a horrendous headache. I carefully followed the doctor's orders. As medical research has progressed, MRI and CAT scans are now available, so these torture tests are no longer performed.

"We don't want to alarm you, but your baby might be retarded," the neurologists told me.

This unpleasant news completely surprised me.

"You carried her while your growth factors were off balance; you had a malfunctioning pituitary gland; and you had problems during the pregnancy," they said.

"Observing my baby from a teacher's viewpoint, I do not agree," I responded in disbelief. "At eleven months, Lisa is putting objects into objects, is already attempting to walk by holding onto furniture, is talking her own language—all the signs

of a very normal infant. I definitely do not agree with you!"
Thankfully, I was right.

Chapter 11

Day of Reckoning

Several days prior to that day, the neurosurgeon, who was going to operate on me, had come to my hospital room, introduced himself and explained the surgical procedure. X-rays or radiographs from the pneumoencephalogram had shown, he told me, that the bones of the sella turcica (which houses the pituitary gland) were bulging with a pituitary tumor. Terms like "pneumoencephalogram" and "sella turcica," might have sounded foreign to me, but tumor was a word I understood, a frightening word.

A mass extended toward the brain, the optic nerves and the carotid artery. The tumor was too large to remove through the nose or the mouth (transphenoidal surgery), so he would perform a craniotomy; that is, he would go in through my skull!

Terribly frightened, "Have you ever performed this type of surgery before?" I asked.

He never answered me and I never questioned whether I should allow him to operate on me. I just accepted the situation. Today, people research extensively to find the very best doctor in a specific field, analyzing both his success ratio and patient recovery statistics. In 1968, we tended to accept whatever our doctors told us, without question. In this instance, I was fortunate in that he turned out to be a leader in his field.

I called Bob at work and told him the surgery date. It had been set for several days away in order for some of the doctors, who wanted to observe, to clear their schedules. I was just so scared and wished that Bob was there with me to hold me. As you can imagine, I spent a lot of time in prayer, talking to my

God.

Because I had taught school and was accustomed to giving presentations, the neurologists asked if I would appear in an auditorium and answer questions before a group of doctors and pre-med students. I agreed. Acromegaly was considered a rare type of pituitary tumor, and any information concerning it, would present an excellent learning experience for both doctors and medical students.

The neurologists also requested that Gracie and I pose for medical pictures to compare our features. We both agreed, but late that night, Gracie called me at the hospital. She was very upset.

"Mary, many of the pictures that I've seen in medical books are in the nude. I will not pose in the nude."

"Neither would I," I responded.

We spoke to the doctors, who assured us that we definitely would be dressed for any pictures that were taken of us.

The presentation in the auditorium went off as planned. Numerous x-rays were mounted on the stage platform and the neurologists, along with the neurosurgeon, discussed the position of the pituitary tumor and the planned point of entry into the skull.

"The patient has a large pituitary tumor; therefore a craniotomy has to be performed. I will be drilling through the skull, removing part of the forehead, the top of the head, and lifting the brain to reach the tumor, which is located behind the eyes," my neurosurgeon said. "Damage can happen to the hypothalamus, which can cause severe shock and trauma to the body through water loss."

Was he trying to frighten me more than I already was, I wondered, as I sat there in my wheelchair listening.

The surgeon continued to discuss other processes of the surgery with medical mumbo jumbo that I did not understand, after which, I was asked to speak about the gradual growth changes that I had experienced in my body over the years.

When I finished, the attendees flooded me with questions. One of the most difficult to answer was: Were you mentally quicker two years ago than you are now?

Two years before, I taught junior high, led discussion groups and gave presentations. It was definitely a different milieu than my recent environment, but mentally slower? I didn't think so.

The attendant wheeled me back to my hospital room after the presentation, and so many different thoughts rambled through my head. From the beginning, I had been extremely worried and frightened about the upcoming surgery, but now, I was just plain scared!

Will I live through the surgery? Will I have a complete recovery or will I be handicapped in some way? Will I be able to hold and hug my baby Lisa? She's so young, only eleven months old. If I don't live, how will she remember me? How difficult is this going to be on Bob...on my parents?

There were no answers. I knew I must trust in the Lord, so I began once again to pray, then, called Bob at work, but I did not want to frighten him with the formidable information I had just heard. I told him as calmly as I could and added how much I wished he were there with me.

He brought Lisa to the hospital that evening, so I could see her playing on the lawn outside my window. We couldn't bring her into the hospital because of the possibility of staff infections, and I couldn't leave; so, we compromised and I watched her from my window and cried. Bob also brought a friend to play with her, while he came into the hospital to hold me and hug me. I needed that so much.

The next day, I called a beautician to come to my hospital room and give me a shampoo, set and styling. In a few days, I would be totally bald, so why not go out in style!

May 22, 1968. The wait was over. Early in the morning in my hospital room, nurses prepared me for surgery, one with a razor in hand, shaving my head. Other nurses stood in the hall, watching. I felt on exhibit, so many people watching me. The nurse put the razor down. I felt my head. Bald. I was baldheaded.

On the appointed day, as I felt my now bald head, Bob, always by my side, encouraged me that everything would be all right.

"You are God's fair-haired child, and He always takes care of you," he reminded me.

An attendant rolled me down the hall on a gurney with Bob walking beside me holding my hand. At the door of the operating room, he bent and kissed me whispering reassurances.

When will I see him again? Will I see him again?

As I went under the anesthetic in the operating room, I prayed for God to direct the surgeon's hands. *God's will be done.* This was my last conscious thought, as the operating room became a blur and darkness set in. It was too late to change my mind.

Later, I was told that the surgery had taken hours, beginning at approximately 7:00 a.m. and lasting till late in the afternoon. One result of acromegaly is that it causes bones to thicken. As a result, the regular drill the surgeon began with could not penetrate my skull, and he had to send out for an air drill. My gynecologist, Dr. Juno, was in the room, observing. Every so often, he stepped out of the room to inform Bob as to the progress of the operation.

My Uncle Ken had come to the hospital to keep Bob Company, as my parents had remained at home to care for Lisa. They felt badly that they could not be there with Bob, but Bob and I were both happy that Lisa was in their capable hands.

When I woke up in the intensive care unit, my whole body felt numb. I slowly opened my eyes, but quickly shut them, turning my head to the side to avoid the bright lights. When I tried again and succeeded in opening them, the light continued to make it difficult to focus. Gradually, shapes came into view...people...and there was Bob! His warm, smiling face just beamed at me.

Thank you, God! I made it!

I immediately experienced an overpowering thirst. The nurse placed a few chips of ice in my mouth.

"Make this last for a while," she said. "You are restricted to liquids and can only have a little bit of ice."

I then learned that my body was severely dehydrated. Many IV's were pumping liquids containing sodium into me. The sodium would help me to retain some of the fluids, because as fast as the fluids entered my body, they exited.

After several hours of limited ice chips, I graduated to one glass of fluid an hour, either a cola or water with sodium. My thirst was so extreme that this was absolute torture. It seems that, due to damage to the pituitary and the hypothalamus caused by the surgery, I had been diagnosed with diabetes insipidus, a problem with water balance in the body, causing great thirst and excessive urination. My body was responding.

In addition to the turban-like bandage that wrapped completely around my head, my appearance was further compromised by my arms, which, due to my body's heavy loss of fluids, looked like those of a 120-year-old hag. My breast tissue, now nothing but wrinkles, lay flat. Lying in the bed in the intensive care unit, I couldn't see my face, which was probably just as well. What the loss of fluids can do to your body, is horrendous.

Bob visited for a short time each hour. When he came into the room in the evening, I pointed to the refrigerator in the corner and tried to convince him to get a can of pop for me. He didn't, of course, knowing that I wasn't supposed to have it, but he told me later that he had taken that as a good sign, since I appeared to be alert and insistent.

I remained in intensive care for several days, while inch-by-inch, my body slowly recovered. My faith gave me great strength during this time. God had brought me this far, I knew he would not leave me now. I prayed a lot during this ordeal, at times, even praying aloud. Being in intensive care, emergencies were commonplace. If I saw an emergency team work on someone, then cover the person's face, and wheel him or her out, I knew that person had died.

"Oh, we moved her up to a room," the nurse would say. I knew that room was the morgue.

Following brain surgery, the patient must be kept awake. Every hour the nurses talked to me to be sure I was not sleeping. The first night after surgery, the neurosurgeon assured me that he was quite positive he had removed the whole tumor. He had taken out most of my pituitary gland, also, which meant, he told me, that I might have to take cortisone for the rest of my life.

This last, fortunately, joined the list of predictions that didn't come true.

"You should not take sleeping pills or birth control pills, because both could affect your pituitary gland, which is already damaged. If you take sleeping pills, you might go up and see your great big Daddy in the sky!" he said. "Watch out, in case a nurse accidentally tries to give you a sleeping pill. Also, with most of your pituitary gland gone, there is no need for you to worry about pregnancy. It won't happen."

What did he mean, "worry" about pregnancy. We had one child, but Bob and I wanted more. He was an only child and he didn't want Lisa to grow up without siblings. This was an unexpected blow.

Each day, I seemed to make progress. My body tissue began to hold fluids, my flesh gradually regained its normal firmness, and I no longer looked like a wrinkled old woman. What a relief! Finally the day came when by the doctor's orders, the attendants moved me from the intensive care unit into a private room. So peaceful! I no longer had to endure the stress and constant activity that went on in the unit. The nursing care there had been excellent with dedicated, optimistic and helpful nurses to watch over me and the other patients. For me, they were really angels of mercy.

"Soon the bandages will come off and you can view my work of art," the neurosurgeon announced on one of his visits. "The incision went from ear to ear across the top of your head. I cut just a quarter of an inch back from your hairline, matching the hairline all the way. I did a very artistic job. Then, I drilled into the skull, removing part of the forehead and the top of the head."

He called it, "a very neat job," also telling me that during the surgery, he had found it necessary to put a metal plate into my head with two metal clips on the right side.

Finally, the day arrived when he removed the turban of bandages.

"Mary, it looks great!" he said and pulled out a large mirror, so I could see his accomplishment.

Looking at it for the first time, I only saw a large bald head with a huge, ugly scar running from one ear to the other. I saw nothing of beauty, but I didn't want to offend him.

"Mary, I drilled through your head with an air drill and you woke up with no headache. Isn't that amazing?"

True. My whole body was reacting in shock to the surgery, but I definitely did not have a headache. As he said, amazing.

The doctor left the bandages off and said that I could shower the next day. I waited for about an hour after he left; then, I headed for the shower.

Water has healing power, and God, I really want to be healed.

I prayed! I showered! For a long time, I stood there enjoying the sensation of the fresh water flowing over my head and cascading down my body. It felt absolutely delicious! No more bandages! Alleluia. What a relief!

My head remained rather numb; however, I experimented and found that if I touched the right side of my head, even though it felt numb, I sensed a tingling or some sort of reaction somewhere else in my head. It felt very strange.

Throughout my recovery, Bob remained his extremely loving, supportive and positive self, constantly there for me. When he arrived in my room and saw my bald head with this big incision running across it, he said, "You look beautiful!"

Beautiful? I didn't see the beauty, but I was grateful to God that I was alive, even with a bald head and an awful scar.

For the next few days, relatives and friends visited me. Not especially pleased with my appearance, I feared my visitors might be offended or even sickened by the sight of the scar; so, I usually placed a hospital white cloth arranged like a scarf on my head.

Besides visiting me in the hospital, Bob continually visited Lisa at my parents' house. Each time he came to see me, he told me about our little daughter and her escapades with Grandma and Grandpa. It gave me great peace of mind to know that Lisa was cared for and loved. Each evening, I thanked God for all the special, wonderful blessings He had given to me, especially the blessing of a wonderful husband, my Bob.

Chapter 12

Home At Last

It was Wednesday, June 5, 1968, only four days before Lisa's birthday, and I was going home! I would be with my baby on her first birthday! Once again, my prayers had been answered.

Embarrassed to have anyone see my bald head, I had asked Bob to bring me a large scarf. Getting dressed and putting the scarf over my head proved to be more exhausting than I had expected. In spite of that, I wanted to stop on the way home to purchase a wig.

The neurosurgeon had warned me that my hair might not grow back. There was no way to predict, he said. Whether it would or not, I still needed a wig for the present. I had looked at myself in the hospital's bathroom mirror and knew that I looked a ghastly, sickly green. I really wanted a wig!

Bob stopped at a nearby Sears store, but before we went in, he pulled out a bag containing some of my hair. When the nurse had cut it all off, he had saved some, anticipating that we would need it to match for a wig. He is remarkable. I wonder if all engineers think like that.

In the wig department, I asked for a private room to try on some wigs.

"Don't be shy," the saleswoman said. "Lots of people have damaged hair. Take off the scarf and let's try some wigs on you."

I insisted on a private room and, when I took off the scarf, she was taken by surprise and realized that I was a bona fide customer for her wigs.

"Oh my God," she said and raced out of the room.

When the saleswoman returned, she had the manager with her. It seems that wigs were going on sale the next week, and the manager offered to sell me a wig at the coming sale price. I really didn't care. I was so tired. All I wanted to do was to get a wig and go home. With the help of the saleswoman, I quickly found one that would do. It didn't match my hair, but it was a reddish-brown color and the right length. I used a handkerchief to protect my incision and placed the wig on my head, happy to have some semblance of a normal look.

We drove home, anticipating that Lisa might not remember me. A friend had told us that when she went into the hospital for only a week, her baby didn't know her when she came home. I had been gone almost a month, but as I stepped from the car, Lisa walked unsteadily toward me, yelling, "Mama! Mama!"

What a fantastic day that was! I had survived the surgery, was home from the hospital, Lisa was walking on her own and she recognized me! I cried, hugged my baby and cried some more. Our family was back together again. *Thank you God! Thank you!*

My parents each hugged me, my mother with tears of thankfulness in her eyes. Looking at Lisa, she said that Gracie and I had been little blonde, blue-eyed girls with still only a little bit of fuzzy hair like Lisa, when we were her age.

As soon as my parents left, I took off the wig. It was heavy on my head and painful, resting as it did on the huge incision across my head. Also, the neurosurgeon had indicated that I should let air get to the incision to help it to heal. Lisa took one look at me, and the look on her little face was one of absolute horror. Immediately, she began to cry and to pull her hair out. It came out in handfuls. We knew seeing me like this would be traumatic for her, but we hadn't expected such a strong reaction. In retrospect, we should have better prepared her, before letting her see Mama bald.

I wanted to let fresh air flow over my incision to continue the healing process, but Lisa continued to pull her hair out. We contacted her pediatrician, who recommended that we shave

Lisa's head; otherwise, she might continue to pull it out for years to come.

Reluctantly, we did as directed, and it was my turn to cry. But now, Lisa looked like Mommy. For days, she continued to look at me and reach for hair that wasn't on her head. She walked around touching and rubbing her head. Finally, she stopped pulling at imaginary hair and, together, within a month or so, we each began to grow some fuzz. I breathed a sigh of relief, knowing we were both going to have hair again.

Before the pituitary surgery, my hair had been thick and coarse in texture. Now, it grew in much thinner than before, but at least I had hair. *Always take a positive outlook about everything.* This was another step on my road to recovery.

Everyday revolved around Lisa, bathing, feeding and playing with her. I still experienced a lot of fatigue, so I enjoyed her three hour nap each afternoon. I could get my own rest then. Bob helped with dinner preparations and he helped enormously with the household chores. He also encouraged me to be patient, to give my body time to heal.

While still in the hospital, it had been decided that I should have a series of radiation treatments in late June and early July. My doctor informed me that the radiation treatments might stop the further growth of any tissue remnants that may have been left in my head from the tumor. I appreciated my neighbor, who offered to baby sit on the days that I went for the radiation treatments. She also had a little girl and the two children played together, while I was gone. I drove to the hospital regularly for several weeks for the treatments, and then discontinued taking the cortisone.

Throughout my stay in the hospital, an endocrinologist had been assigned to my case, and upon my leaving the hospital, he became my internist and family doctor as well. He was a cute young doctor with a high interest in my medical problems. Over the years, this fantastic doctor has pulled me out of many emergency situations. He was another of my blessings from God.

Recovery after my brain surgery came quicker than I expected. The first sign of recovery appeared within a matter of weeks, when my visual fields returned to normal. I noticed one day that when I entered a room, while looking straight ahead, I could also see the sides of the room. Most people take that peripheral vision for granted, but for me, its return was exciting. Now, driving a car would be much safer.

During my stay in the hospital, the doctors mentioned that they did not know if my menstrual cycle would resume as normal, or if it might begin as though I were at the puberty stage and last much longer, or it could stop completely. So, my next sign of recovery occurred, when in August of 1968, I had a normal menstrual period. To me, this was truly a sign that I was on the road back to normality. Meanwhile, other changes had occurred: no more lactation, no more severe headaches with flashing lights, no more nausea and no more dizziness.

During this recovery period, a new problem began to surface. I had felt extreme fatigue for many, many years, but now the fatigue was different. It had happened after Lisa's birth and was happening again, after surgery. The fatigue I now experienced was accompanied by an emotional problem that I did not understand.

I continually felt like crying. I was extremely emotionally upset, and I had no idea why. Little incidents that normally would never have bothered me became monumental problems. Tears flowed freely. Fortunately, Bob recommended that I bring this problem to my endocrinologist's attention. Meeting with him, I explained how frustrated I was with myself because of these sudden explosive outbursts, with tears and anger, over situations that never should have disturbed me.

"Mary, that is normal," my doctor reassured me in his usual calm manner. "It's a physical weakness. Your body is tired. You are experiencing a lot of fatigue as you recover from surgery and this physical weakness shows itself emotionally. When it displays itself after the birth of a child, as it did after Lisa was born, it's called, post-partum depression. Let the tears flow; just understand it for what it is. "

I was not a psycho or a neurotic. I was normal! Just hearing the doctor say it, calmed me. I hoped and prayed that Bob would understand and be able to continue to cope with the emotional roller coaster I was on; although, I don't know why I worried about that. He seemed to always adjust to every situation as it happened. He said that was just part of being in love.

Forgive me for being repetitive, but over the years, two things have helped me to fight depression, loneliness and fear. I have always had a positive attitude about life, and most of all, I have always maintained a strong faith in my God, Who always has taken care of me.

During the next few months of recovery, Bob was always there for me, helpful in every way, thankful that I was improving, and making it possible for me to enjoy my time with Lisa.

Chapter 13

Something's Moving Inside

The beautiful fall weather of October and November arrived and my health had improved so much that I handled most of the household work, preparing the meals and setting out bowls of autumn flowers, but not scrubbing floors or cleaning windows.

After operating on my brain, my neurosurgeon had told me, "With most of your pituitary gland gone, there is no need for you to worry about pregnancy. It won't happen." I had been upset with this news, but why then in December, just a few months later, had my menstrual periods stopped? Could he have been wrong? Was I pregnant?

I made an appointment with my gynecologist and took a pregnancy test, which was negative. Then, I made an appointment with my neurosurgeon. Afraid that the pituitary tumor was growing again, my neurosurgeon decided on a return to radiation therapy, which I began in early January.

Still experiencing constant fatigue, now I also had to deal with nausea, which often is associated with radiation therapy.

Knowing that I would need help and someone to care for baby Lisa, Bob and I decided to sell the new home we had just built and move closer to my parents. Until that could happen, each morning, I drove across town to drop Lisa off with my parents and then took the long, exhausting drive to the hospital for my treatments. Fortunately, my neighbor offered to watch Lisa once in a while, which gave me some relief. I was also grateful for Lisa's long afternoon naps.

We were able to sell our brick ranch house quickly and contracted to build a new colonial style house just a few miles from my parents' house. It would be completed around Christmas 1969, about eight months away.

Every month, I was given a pregnancy test by my gynecologist and each month, it was negative.

Five days a week throughout January, February, March and April, I received radiation therapy. Taking me by elevator down to what appeared to be a huge auditorium, the radiologist daily placed me on a table, positioned weights at the sides of my head and poised the radiation machine above me.

"Don't move during the treatment, or you could have your brain zapped," she warned me each time.

Scary words. Of course, I didn't move. Who would? As usual, I prayed a great deal. The technician left me alone in the room, while she watched me on closed-circuit television. Each time, when it was over, she accompanied me back upstairs in the elevator. The procedure never varied.

My hair, though thinner than before, had grown quite long. The radiologist had an unpleasant message for me.

"Don't be surprised if your hair should suddenly fall out in clumps. Your scalp will be just like your face, nice and smooth," she said. "Lengthy radiation therapy can cause that to happen."

Meanwhile, the nausea and fatigue continued. Spring was coming with warmer weather, but it held no joy for me. I was so depressed. My hair was about to fall out; I had a fatigue problem again; I was nauseous; I was making an arduous drive to the hospital five days a week, every week; and it seemed that the tumor was coming back.

One day, as I walked from the parking area to the hospital entrance, workmen up on the building started catcalling and whistling. That really perked me up and brightened my day. I needed to know I was still attractive. Thank you, gentlemen; you did more than just make my day. I really did feel better.

I told my beautician that my hair might fallout. I didn't want her to be disturbed, if it began to fall out while she was combing it. The Saturday before Easter, I wanted an attractive hairdo, something like a twist. My beautician did a great job. "It's absolutely gorgeous," she said, admiring her handiwork. I was delighted.

The morning after Easter, I woke up to find hair all over my pillow. I cried and took out the wig. This time, I had no problems with Lisa. I wasn't totally bald, only on the sides going up to the crown.

The radiation treatments continued until May, when I notified my doctors that, "There is something moving inside me. It's either a tapeworm or a baby, but I feel a fluttering."

The faces of the radiologists showed surprise, then disbelief. They decided to continue the radiation treatments anyway, but now placed a heavy lead covering over my chest and abdomen, which they had not done before. I was so skinny, with no visual signs of a pregnancy, and, as usual, the test turned out to be negative. I now know that a pregnancy test would have been negative even at nine months. I guess my body just doesn't know how to follow the rules and kill the rabbits.

Finally, in the middle of May, my gynecologist informed me that I was, indeed, pregnant. Bob had been predicting that for some time, based on my emotional state. The radiologists wanted to finish the series of treatments, and my gynecologist began to make some serious recommendations.

"I won't do the abortion myself, but a doctor friend of mine will handle it," he told me, assuming that we would agree to an abortion. "No way can you expect the baby to be normal," he continued. "Have an abortion."

The neurosurgeon agreed, saying that with most of my pituitary gone, the exhaustion problems that I had, plus the acromegaly, I definitely should consider an abortion.

Bob and I never questioned what we would do. If this was our love child, we would love it. Each child is a gift from God. Never would we consider aborting our baby. In fact, we were happy! Now we knew for sure that my problems were definitely not caused by a return of the brain tumor. We decided that there are some times in life when you must leave everything in God's hands and prayed for a healthy baby.

Because of the original confusion, I had a short pregnancy. My due date was calculated to be October 2, 1969. During that four-and-a-half months, we were on another roller coaster. We worried; we prayed; we were excited; we were scared. This miracle baby was from God, and we knew He would give us strength.

I felt great during the pregnancy just knowing the brain tumor was not coming back. The nausea stopped, but the fatigue continued. Because of my pituitary problem, Lisa had been born by a caesarean section and my gynecologist knew this one had to be a C-section too. We asked our pediatrician to be there to check the baby immediately.

"You have an absolutely perfect baby boy," the pediatrician said to reassure us, as soon as the baby was lifted from me.

Dark haired Eric Stevens, looking like Bob, weighed in at six pounds seven ounces. What great joy we felt! This was our miracle baby! We were so blessed, and I was so happy that in my usual fashion, I screamed my delight.

Bob's mother's birthday had been October 2. Eric was born on his grandmother's birthday. I wish I had known her and that she had lived to see her grandchildren.

I was in better physical shape for Eric's birth than I had been for Lisa's, but due to my fatigue syndrome, the doctor would not allow me to breast-feed him. That was a disappointment, as it had been with Lisa; but, at least with Eric, I was able to hold him to give him his bottle. What a joy!

The doctors were so proud of the birth of our baby, against all odds. The neurosurgeon said it was because of his great skill; the radiologists said they did it; but, my husband was right when he said, "I did it."

"Yes, along with a great deal of help from the Lord," I commented.

The neurosurgeons repeated the same old statement. "This won't happen again. Don't worry; you had most of your pituitary removed, so you won't get pregnant again." This time I ignored them.

Three months later, we moved into our new house, near my parents' home. Here we were our family all together. We had ourselves, our two beautiful children, and Buddy, our black Labrador retriever. *Thank you, God!*

What was it the neurosurgeons had said? I wouldn't get pregnant again? When Eric was six months old, my menstrual periods stopped. Of course, the pregnancy test was negative and, of course, we knew I was pregnant again. Bob said that I could never keep my pregnancies a secret from him, even if I wanted to. My emotional state would always give me away.

During this pregnancy, the fetus frightened us; it was quiet, hardly ever moving. Both my other babies had been active. To make it worse, the doctor had difficulty hearing a heartbeat; it was so faint. The due date for the C-section was May twenty-fourth. I worried. I prayed.

As usual, my worrying was unnecessary. Gina weighing just over six pounds, was a perfect little baby girl. The quietness she displayed before birth followed her into her life. A happy, bubbly baby, she loved a schedule and went right to sleep at nap or night time. Our quiet, gentle baby Gina has grown into a quiet, gentle adult.

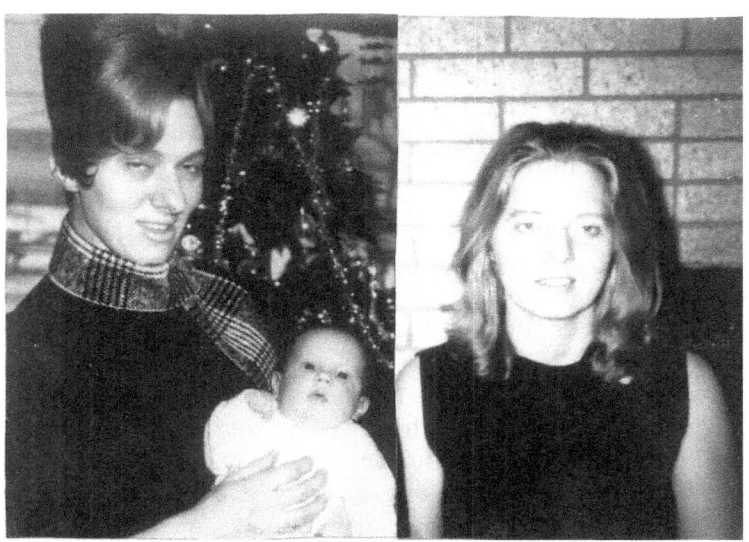

Christmas 1969. Mary is on the left and Gracie on the right. A year and a half after surgery, Mary still has the large hang lip, larger lips, a wider jowl, jutting jaw, larger nose, higher, more pronounced cheek bones, drooping eyelids and large hands—all signs of acromegaly. Mary is holding Eric, her "miracle baby," who is almost three months old. Mary is wearing a wig.

My brain had been operated on successfully, but I still had acromegaly. It is a chronic disease and accounted for my continued fatigue to the point of exhaustion. After Gina's birth, my exhaustion took the form of night sweating. Frequently, our bed sheets and blanket were totally soaked. I'd wake in the middle of the night, wet with perspiration. I'd dry off and then Bob and I would change the sheets. Poor Bob. We sometimes were up and down all night. He wouldn't let me get up to fix a bottle for the new baby. He said that was his time with his little daughter.

With two little ones, Bob and I could each dress one, carry them to the car, go shopping or do whatever was necessary. Now with three, it wasn't that easy. On our first trip out after Gina was born, I dressed Lisa and carried her out to the car and Bob dressed Eric and carried him to the car. We got in and drove about a half block, looked at each other and hurried back to the house. We had forgotten Gina. Fortunately, we found her sleeping peacefully in her bassinet. That never happened again!

Other women take care of their homes and their children and survive. I could have too, if it hadn't been for the extreme fatigue that I continued to suffer.

"I didn't marry you to clean the house. I married you to be my wife, so let's get a cleaning woman," Bob finally said.

With Barbara's arrival, my world changed. I began to feel like a real person. I didn't feel obligated to do household chores. Months before, the neurosurgeon had mentioned to Bob that I could probably shop for hours and do fine, but the exertion of scrubbing a floor might be too much. We both knew from experience that those were true words. During my children's early years, I enjoyed many fun activities with them, taking them to parks, to friends' houses, to the library, and directing them in many learning activities at home. What an understanding husband!

Barbara became an integral part of our household. She cleaned the house each week and knew how to manipulate the children. She promised them that if they put away their toys, she would let them help her clean the house. Her technique worked. She knew how much I depended on her and the effort she put forth, and I appreciated it.

Barbara remained with us for about seven years. What a fantastic person! She was truly one of my blessings from God.

Chapter 14

I Saw the Light

Allergic reactions to almost everything became my next big problem. They began with the CAT scans that the doctors ordered to monitor a possible return of the tumor. After the first few scans, my body began to swell and ugly blotches broke out on my skin. I was reacting to the dye. Resolution: CAT scans without dye.

One day, a year or so later, during dinner in a local restaurant, I became violently ill and my throat felt thick and swollen. Bob called the health department to report that I had eaten rancid food. Not so. I had developed an allergy to fish and all types of seafood, including some of my favorites: lobster, shrimp and crab.

The reactions came swiftly. I could no longer take penicillin or eat eggs.

Why? Were these reactions to the pituitary surgery? To damage to the pituitary and hypothalamus from radiation? Was my immune system compromised? There were no answers.

Later in the year, after taking a prescribed antibiotic and a painkiller in advance of a root canal, I went into extreme dehydration, turning stiff with severe pain throughout the back of my head, which I couldn't bend, and my spine. In addition, I couldn't stop urinating or vomiting.

Bob called a babysitter, wrapped me in a blanket and rushed me to a nearby emergency room. Incredibly, they didn't want me as a patient, because of my medical history. They called my endocrinologist and arranged for my transfer to another hospital, where he was on the staff. They said they were not even going to bill me. They didn't even want me on their records!

"We think you'll make it to the next hospital," one of the doctors said to me, as they readied me for the transfer. Not a comforting thought.

A team of doctors awaited me and worked on me all night, until my condition stabilized. They gave me spinal taps and tested for spinal meningitis, encephalitis, even leptospirosis because I owned a dog! The diagnosis: severe allergic reaction to a painkiller and an antibiotic.

The next day after being admitted to the hospital, a nurse came into my room with a cup of medication. Because it didn't look like the medicine that I normally took, I questioned her.

"The doctor probably ordered a change in your meds," she snapped. "Here, take it!"

I did, and quickly realized that I'd made a big mistake. I felt sick and asked the patient in the other bed to call my husband and my doctor and tell them what had happened, as I rushed into the bathroom. When the doctor arrived, we had to go through the whole stabilizing procedure, because I was dehydrating again.

Since then, I have been extremely cautious about any medication given to me in a hospital. My doctor said that he would personally notify me of any changes he might make and told me to call him if I had any questions in this regard. Often in the hospital, I did my own charting for input and output of fluids. When the numbers indicated that I had returned to normal, I called my doctor, day or night, in order to be released.

As my allergic reactions increased, we made many such rushed visits to the emergency room. I could depend on my endocrinologist to always be there for me. If I were ill at home, he even called in the evening to check on my condition.

These medical emergencies were difficult for my children. Often, without warning, I disappeared from their lives to spend days hospitalized. They and Bob must have gone through much turmoil during these uncertain times.

My allergies led to problems that other people didn't have. It was our habit to take a two week vacation on a lake in Oscoda each year. At one cabin, the septic tank backed up into the shower. Most people would have felt a little revolted, a little sickly. I dehydrated. Back to the hospital. Another time, we stayed in a cabin that had been cleaned before our arrival, but, apparently, not clean enough for me. Surprise! Dehydration again and back to the hospital.

We soon learned that we had to take extra precautions. The burden fell on Bob. When we first arrived at any cottage, I went to town to shop and Bob cleaned the cabin.

The same was true for restaurants. If a restaurant appeared to be dirty or greasy, we drove on to another one. Often, we stopped at several before finding one that was acceptable. Our lifestyle revolved around my health problems. I didn't like it, but that's the way it had to be.

When Gina, our youngest child, began attending preschool, we made another major decision. We decided to move to Rochester Hills in an attempt to improve the children's educational opportunities. After a short stint of house-hunting, we found a lovely home with a treed setting in Christian Hills, which we bought and moved into.

With all three children in school, I had time on my hands. I definitely did not want to sit home alone, watching someone else clean my house. I needed something to do. With my health still precarious, I knew I couldn't return to the rigorous schedule of teaching. I needed a career that would allow me some flexibility and decided that becoming a Realtor might just be the right job for me. I began attending classes.

It proved to be a good decision. I went on to have a successful career. Throughout the eighties, I won free trips for my high sales, even though I still experienced a lot of fatigue. I could arrange my schedule to suit my needs for rest. In time, I volunteered to teach sessions for the local Board of Realtors. These sessions addressed some of the problems of the day that concerned me: fair housing, discrimination and other educational programs required for new Realtors.

During this time, we took the children to Disneyland. When passing through the security check station at the airport, I set off the alarms. I realized that the metal in my head had to be the culprit. What a surprise! Shortly after the surgery in 1968, my forehead had begun to appear damaged. I grew bangs to cover the spot. At the airport, I raised my bangs and showed them my dented forehead.

"I have metal in my head."

The attendant passed me through. The children thought that was great!

This kind of thing happened many times over the years, when we traveled. Each time I made the alarm go off, the kids would say, "There goes Mom!" In those days, I only had to lift my bangs and tell the security guard about my metal plate. Today, that might not be enough.

One of the most memorable experiences of my life occurred in the mid-seventies. A dentist gave me a Novocain injection prior to filling a cavity. Suddenly, I couldn't blink. My eyes and the top of my head were frozen, but not the nerve in my tooth. When he drilled, the pain was excruciating, and my head and eyes remained frozen for hours. Since the action of blinking brings moisture to the eyes, my eyes became dry and I had to use a suction cup to remove my contacts that night.

Thinking that he must have hit the wrong nerve, I returned to this dentist for a root canal. I told him what had happened the last time, but he ignored it and injected Novocain again. This time, I immediately felt weird, beginning to feel very cold.

I tried to call out to the dentist to help me, but no words came out; all the screaming was inside me. I got colder and colder. It was a coldness that really hurt. *When will the dentist notice that there is something wrong with me?*

I became so cold, I couldn't feel myself anymore; then, I felt nothing.

I started traveling backwards very rapidly through a dark tunnel, and began to feel warmth surrounding me. I left the tunnel and floated in a beautiful, warm white light out in space, way up in the sky. The light seemed to penetrate into my whole being. The scenario was so peaceful, so fantastic, and so beautiful, words fail to describe it.

I felt that if I turned, I would be absorbed into the light. I sensed that there were people behind me, but I did not turn to look at them or at the light. Instead, I looked down at myself in the dentist's chair.

I saw my car in the parking lot, the traffic in the street, and I could see through the roof of the building and look down at myself, limp in the dentist's chair. I saw my dentist and his associate, along with the dental assistant working over me, frantically trying to give me oxygen. They worked for some time, and I could hear everything they said.

"We've lost her. She's dead!" my dentist said.

Shaking their heads in disbelief, they left me–my body–alone, still sunken in the chair, and walked down a narrow hallway to an office. They were very quiet.

I knew I was dead. I felt absolutely no fear. The moment was so enticing and so peaceful, but I knew I still had work to do. I wanted to raise my three children; so, I began talking to God. The words came tumbling out.

"God, I must go back! I'm not finished. I still have work to do. I have my three children to raise. You must let me go back!"

Gradually, I began to move downward toward the tunnel. At the same time, I felt a tinge of cold. I knew then that God was going to allow me to go back. The coldness became stronger and stronger, as I quickly began sliding downward into the tunnel and into my body. The coldness was replaced by body warmth.

When I came to my senses, and was able to function, I called out to the dentists, still in the other room.

"Help! Doctor, I need your help!

My dentist rushed into the room. "We already pronounced you dead."

"I know. I heard you. I was watching everything you did–from way up in the sky."

My dentist seemed quite disturbed. He wanted to call for medical help or for my husband, but I persuaded him to wait. I stayed in the chair until I was steady enough to walk. I assured the dentist that I could drive myself home and I did. I was positively all right.

What I learned from that experience, I will remember for the rest of my life. I am not as fearful of death, as I was before. I would never pursue death, because I believe that time and moment are for God to determine. People often say they don't want to be alone when they die. I agree that to have relatives near you, talking with you at the time of your death sounds great; but I learned that when your body begins to shut down and you go into shock due to the rapid drop of body temperature, you are alone with God. Even if your relatives are in the room with you, they cannot help you. You may appear to be in a coma or even dead to those around you, but your mind is active and able to communicate with the only One Who is important in your life at that time—God!

In the months to come, my dentist attempted to hypnotize me in order to control the pain, but it didn't work. He had taken classes in dental hypnosis and really wanted to succeed. I wanted it to work also. I certainly didn't want the pain; but I couldn't relax enough to let someone else control my life. Staying in control of my life has always been dominant with me; but the dentist was frustrated with me.

"You must not be too intelligent; otherwise, you would cooperate and let me hypnotize you! You just aren't cooperative."

In the ensuing months, I had dental work done without anesthesia of any kind. The pain was intense and my facial muscles contorted for days afterward.

"Why don't you try getting drunk?" my dentist asked. "At least, your facial muscles would be more relaxed, even though you would still feel the pain."

I put off the inevitable until I had no choice. The tooth hurt badly and my gum had begun to swell up.

I had never been drunk and I knew I couldn't allow myself to become totally drunk. Perhaps, I could drink enough alcohol so that I would be more relaxed. I didn't want to do it at home. I contacted a restaurant in Rochester and explained my problem to them. They agreed to open the bar area at nine a.m., just for me. This was really something different! I asked some of my Realtor friends to join me in getting drunk for a good cause. Several of them showed up. They thought it was funny.

I didn't want to consume a heavy volume of alcohol, or I

would become nauseous.

"When I begin to feel really light-headed and happy, but not totally drunk, I will give you a signal and we can leave for the dentist's office," I told Bob.

Amid a lot of laughter and jokes, I drank two strong pina coladas, followed by boisterous waving, cheering and good luck wishes from my friends, as Bob and I left the bar to drive to the dentist's office.

It was all for nothing. As soon as the dentist began to drill on the tooth, I began to scream. The dentist sang "Jesus Christ, Superstar" in a loud voice, attempting to drown out my yelling.

Afterward, laughingly I told him, "I was screaming because I can't stand your singing."

For several years, I called various allergists to ask if they tested for antibiotics and painkillers. They all said, no; until I finally found the allergist who caused great positive changes in my life.

This short, doctor with grayish brown hair and a long white medical coat that flared out whenever he turned around looked like an escapist from Disneyland. He was a human, walking, medical dictionary, full of energy and enthusiasm.

"Mary, you are a challenge to the medical profession, and I am excited to have you as my patient," he said. "Doctors sometimes wait a lifetime to find a patient like you."

I also felt excited, but for a different reason. Here, at last, was a doctor who believed me and wanted to help me. He tested me for painkillers and, while ruling out Novocain, xylocaine, marcaine and others, he found that I reacted well to carbocaine. He also found several antibiotics that were acceptable. Over time, I developed allergies even to some of these, but for a short time, I could take them.

Luckily, I also located a dentist who would work on my teeth in the emergency room of a local hospital. Worried that I might develop an allergy to carbocaine, he decided to do root canals on several of my teeth before that could happen. The front teeth that I had broken as a child were prime candidates. This was a great relief to me, even though I have not yet developed an allergy to that painkiller. In fact, I carried carbocaine with me for years, in case of an emergency, since many hospitals and doctors didn't stock this drug.

The allergist tested me for such things as food and mold. I followed his suggestion to stop eating certain foods and, although I found that they were not the cause of my repeated bouts with diarrhea or of my headaches, they were causing me to be drowsy and sleepy. When I stopped eating them, my energy level increased.

I wondered: *How many students have I taught who appeared to be listless or lethargic, and who might really have had a food allergy?* Something to seriously consider.

I developed allergies to so many foods: tomatoes, strawberries, apples, bananas, berries. The only fruits that I can eat are grapes, pears and hard oranges, without attacks of severe cramping and diarrhea, usually accompanied by shock. The attacks lasted for several days and other foods to which I was not normally allergic, caused the same reaction during that time.

My family continually adjusted to my allergies. The children ordered special pizza with no tomato, double cheese and mushrooms for me. It was good and, when friends came over, everyone wanted to try my pizza. We had to watch them, or none would be left for me.

I was saddened to learn after my earlier brain surgery that none of the doctors could predict if there would ever be a reversal to the abnormal growth changes I had experienced. You will remember that my nose had become enlarged; as had my lips and a hang lip had developed among other unpleasant changes.

Beginning in the seventies and extending into the eighties, I happily noted gradual facial and bodily changes taking place. My teeth changed from a protruding jaw to a large over-bite, to a cross-bite, to being edge to edge. Ear aches and pain in the back section of my lower jaw were the results of adjustments to my jaw area. The dentist suggested braces or cracking my jaw during these changes, but I assured him neither was necessary.

Tissue changes in my face continued over the years and my nose gradually became smaller. My lips and hang lip lessened until they finally returned to normal. The large jowl and high cheeks receded and shrank and my coarse, thick facial skin softened, along with the acne on my shoulders disappearing. My feet began to lose pads of skin. I know how a snake feels, because I literally shed my skin. The progress was slow and I used nail files and pumice stones to help it along. By the late seventies, my shoe size had gone from a D to a B width. This made buying shoes much easier.

The doctors did not expect a change in the size of the bones that house the pituitary gland, but when the radiologist superimposed my CAT scans, he discovered that they were indeed reduced.

My allergy problems continued and, as usual, the reactions were severe. Relief would come and then something else would cause another reaction and the whole process would be repeated. Such care had to be taken with my meal preparations. My chicken could not be roasted in the same oven with potatoes. On holidays, I could make a delicious stuffing for our guests, but I couldn't eat it. I developed a philosophy: *So, I have allergies, but I am still alive!*

In the early eighties, my eyelids began to droop; a problem caused by the acromegaly. In time, they drooped so much that they interfered with my vision. My ophthalmologist recommended surgery to shorten the eyelids. I thought a plastic surgeon should be called in, but the ophthalmologist said that he had performed many of this type of operation.

I told him about my allergies to antibiotics and painkillers. He rolled his eyes in obvious disbelief. He also didn't believe me, when I told him that any medications had to be approved by my allergist, but he reluctantly did so. I was awake during the surgery and heard him make a remark to the doctor assisting him.

"This patient has bad allergies, but wait until she finds out she has damaged lungs."

This upset me and I spoke up, "My blood pressure was probably 110 over 70 when I came into this hospital, and it will probably be the same when I leave, but right now, it must be quite high. I've had a scar tissue problem in my lungs since the early seventies," I continued, "and it is definitely not a problem. This is not the time or place to discuss a possible lung problem."

As a teacher, I gave this doctor a failing grade in diplomacy. As for the surgery, he did a sloppy job, and I added him to the list of doctors that I would never go back to again.

After the surgery, I could no longer wear contact lens. The scar tissue under my eyelids would be an irritant. Within months, I began to show an allergy to eye makeup, both eye liner and mascara–a real problem for a woman! I tried several hypo-allergenic types of eye makeup, but every time, the skin around my eyes became heavily inflamed, taking days for the swelling to go down. Finally, I gave up and have not worn eye makeup since. To make it worse, my skin became more sensitive to certain soaps, shampoos, perm solutions and other types of lotion, so I had to exercise extreme caution when using any of these products. *What would happen next?*

Chapter 15

Water Poured Down

One day in the eighties, Bob and I attended a friend's house party. I didn't feel well. I ate nothing and drank only a glass of pop. At home later that night, when I walked into our bedroom, the room began to spin. I was spinning in circles, couldn't walk, breathing heavily. *What's happening to me?* I screamed for Bob. He quickly got the children into bed, carried me out to the car and rushed me to the hospital emergency room.

Once assured I was not on drugs, the doctors gave me shots of Dramamine. They started IV's and extensive testing, but the results were inconclusive. Because of my experience of being given the wrong medication in the hospital, I didn't want to stay there. I wanted to go home, but I still couldn't walk. Bob helped me into a wheelchair, wheeled me out to the car, drove home and carried me back up to the bedroom. By now, it was eight o'clock in the morning.

When the children woke up, Bob explained what had happened and drove the girls to the babysitter's house. Eric chose to go down the street to play with his friend, Jim. Bob left me on the bed with a phone nearby. The spinning had stopped, but I still couldn't walk.

Jill, a neighbor, whom I did not know at this time, was out jogging. When she started to pass by Jim's house, she stopped, went up the walk and rang the doorbell.

When Jim's mother, opened the door, Jill said, "I don't know why, but something told me to ring your doorbell. I just sensed there might be a problem. Is anything wrong?"

"No problem here, but Eric's mom is sick, and Eric is very worried about her."

"God must want us to pray with her," Jill said.

So, Doris, Jim's mom, called me and asked if she and Jill could come over and pray with me. Almost before I could answer, they were walking down the street. They came up to my bedroom and together we prayed silently for healing. After a short time, I praised God aloud.

"Thank you, God! I feel like the roof of the house is open above me and water is pouring down. It feels like rain is coming right through the roof of the house. I just know God is answering our prayers for healing."

Immediately, I stood up and thanked the women profusely for coming in and praying with me. I repeated that it felt like water pouring down on me. "I know it's a blessing from God and I am healed."

I hugged them both, walked them to the door, and thanked them again for coming. After they left, I took a shower. Now water was really pouring down on me and I loved the feeling of it. Then, I did what every mother does, I cleaned up the kitchen.

I explained what had happened to a completely surprised Bob when he came home.

"I believe you, absolutely," he said.

Within the hour the phone rang. It was the emergency room nurse.

"You must come back into the hospital immediately. The tests indicate an emergency situation."

I asked what the problem was and she said that my potassium level was so low, that I couldn't function.

"Can it change by itself in a matter of hours?" I asked.

"No, definitely not."

I told her that I had recovered and would call my family doctor. I told my endocrinologist what had happened and he also believed me.

"Are you sure you're okay, now?"

"I'm fine."

He asked me to come into his office the next day, so he could run some of the tests again. I did and the test results showed all normal levels. *Thank you, God*

Unfortunately, my allergies to medicine continued to worsen. In addition, the tests were no longer producing accurate results. In order to determine my reactions, my allergist now had to give me some of a medication and have me wait in his office for a few hours for observation. By this method, he discovered that I could take the antibiotic cleosin, but only by mouth. It wasn't much, but it was something.

The family needed another change. In the early eighties, Bob and I decided our house in Christian Hills was too small for us. Lisa, a teenager, needed more privacy, we thought. She needed to have her own bedroom.

The family voted in answer to the question: Do you want to move to another neighborhood or add on to this house?

Bob and all three children voted to stay, so we planned a large addition to the house. We added 1,650 square feet plus a new basement to an existing 2,400 square foot house, making it into a contemporary multi-level. This all happened because we needed one more bedroom!

Chapter 16

More Brain Surgery

The children, of course, knew that I had health problems. How could they not? But, when they were in their early teens, Bob and I gathered them together and explained in detail most of the problems that had beset me, and the physical changes that occurred over the years because of acromegaly, the brain surgery, the radiation that both Eric and I had in the sixties, the recommendation for an abortion for Eric, which we refused, and how blessed we have all been by God.

When Eric was sixteen, some of his friends recommended that he apply for a modeling position at J-Board, a promotional division of Jacobson's in Rochester, a high fashion retail store. Eric was hired and became involved in both formal and informal modeling, including runway modeling for ski clothes and suits–modeling in the mall areas. Eric was handsome; mothers have the right to say those things.

His graduation from high school was held at Meadowbrook Hall. At the end of the graduation ceremony, Eric suddenly hovered over me, and then gave me a big hug.

"Mom, thanks for choosing to have me!"

Emotionally touched by his words, I cried.

Not having him had never been an option for me. I realized what we would have missed had our decision been any different.

In the late eighties, I began to have more headaches and a recurrence of the dizziness deep within my head. Often, I closed my eyes and shook my head, hoping the dizziness would clear up. It didn't happen.

My forehead looked distorted from the damage done to it by the surgery in 1968. There was a small hole between my forehead bones. It appeared to be sunken. Now, my forehead began to swell with a large, protruding lump that was quite painful. I also experienced pressure around my right eye.

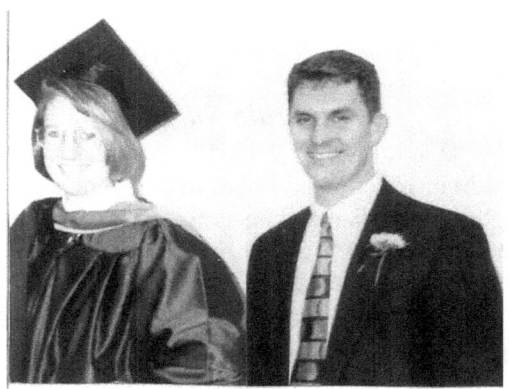

Lisa and Eric

At this time, all of our three children were in college. Lisa, definitely not retarded, was at Western Michigan, majoring in two undergraduate degrees–environmental sciences: biology and English. She went on for a master's degree in environmental

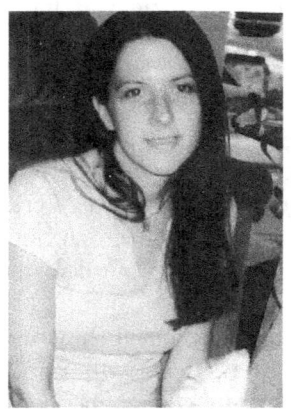

Gina

hydrogeology. Eric, definitely normal, was at Michigan State, getting a degree in sociology, majoring in criminal justice; and Gina was at Central Michigan, aiming for a Bachelor of Arts degree. We spent a great deal of time visiting university campuses.

My real estate career had slowed down tremendously. All this pain in my head worried me that the pituitary tumor might be returning. Something seemed to be growing both inside and outwardly in my forehead.

In 1990, I was referred to another neurosurgeon, because my previous doctor had retired. The new doctor had to be a participant in our health insurance program. At the same time, I researched and found the retired neurosurgeon who had operated on me in 1968. I phoned him.

"Do you remember me, Mary Stevens? You operated on me in 1968 for acromegaly." I said. "I'd like to meet with you for lunch and personally thank you for the great job you did."

"Of course, I remember you, and I'd love to meet you for lunch."

A few days later, we met in a quaint little restaurant of his choice.

His first words to me were, "Mary, I'm surprised you're still alive. We never expected you would live this long."

This left me a bit shaken.

During a meeting with my new neurosurgeon, he remarked that the swelling that was growing quite rapidly in my forehead might be eating through the bone. I thought about that sunken hole in my forehead, which created an opening into the skull.

"We will schedule you for an MRI immediately," the doctor said.

"No, I thought I couldn't have an MRI, since I have metal in my head."

"That really doesn't matter. You must have an MRI."

When I arrived for the test, the radiologist asked, "Mrs. Stevens, do you have any metal in your head?"

"Yes, I have enough metal in my head to set off alarms in airports."

Mary J. Stevens

"We could fry your brain! This is a mistake. Your doctor should never have ordered an MRI for you," the radiologist exclaimed.

I called the neurosurgeon and repeated the radiologist's remarks to him. I was angry and worried. Time was of the essence. My forehead was swelling and the pain was more intense and, now, we had to wait a few more weeks for the results of a dyeless CAT scan.

As soon as the results of the CAT scan were available, surgery was scheduled for the following week. It was June 1990.

The point of entry for the surgery was directly into the forehead, just above the right eye. You can't imagine how relieved I was that the lab results showed it was not cancer, but within a month of the surgery, the pain returned. The bone was also swelling and the same old dizziness and pressure deep within my head returned. The surgeon had not removed all the growth.

"Didn't you scrape the inside portion of the bone for remnants of the tumor?" I asked.

"I didn't have enough operating time," was the surgeon's response.

My confidence in him was shaken. By early fall, another surgery had been scheduled. This time, a bone would be removed and reconstructive work would be done on my forehead. A plastic surgeon would assist the neurosurgeon.

The plastic surgeon's schedule was heavy and I had to wait for three weeks for an appointment. Not wanting to leave anything to chance, I called his office and asked if he did, indeed, do facial reconstructive surgery. It was fortunate that I made that call or another three weeks would have been wasted.

I spoke to the doctor's receptionist, who relayed my question to him.

"The doctor says, definitely not, Mrs. Stevens. He recommends that if you want the best man for the job, you should contact Dr. Vasileff in Birmingham."

In order for the insurance company to pay for the surgery, a plastic surgeon must be referred by a neurosurgeon.

"The plastic surgeon you referred me to says he does not

104

specialize in reconstructive surgery. He recommends a Dr. Vasileff in Birmingham. He said that Dr. Vasileff is excellent, the very best. Will you refer me to him, so my insurance will pay for the necessary surgery?"

"Yes, go ahead and make the appointment with Dr. Vasileff," the neurosurgeon responded. Later, I regretted not getting this statement in writing!

The neurosurgeon wanted the point of entry to be in the forehead and the surgery limited to that area. The plastic surgeon insisted that total reconstruction be done, meaning a full craniotomy with an incision from ear to ear across the center top of the head. They would remove the metal plate and metal clips along with any tumors they might find. Finally, they would insert the metal plate and clips along with various forms of plastics, including plastic bones for my forehead.

The plastic surgeon prevailed and the operation was scheduled for Friday, November 2, 1990. It took longs hours and, again, I prayed to God to direct the surgeons' hands.

I had told Dr. Vasileff that I was tired of wearing wigs, so he obligingly left a quarter of an inch of hair around my face and left the back portion of my head unshaved. I would be able to wear a scarf, instead of a wig. What a fantastic doctor!

This surgery differed from that of 1968 in that they did not have to touch the pituitary and the incision was farther back, across the center of my head. Without the pituitary area involved, I had no dehydration problems this time.

Dr. Vasileff stopped to see me after the operation.

"The surgery was more involved that I had projected," he said. "Therefore, my bill to the insurance company will be higher than anticipated. There will be no additional charge to you, and if the insurance company refuses to pay the higher bill, there still will be no additional charge to you."

"During the surgery," he added, "I removed the scar tissue on the underside of the incision that was made on you back in 1968. Now, your hair will grow back thicker in that area."

I couldn't ask for a better doctor, and, by the way, the insurance company did pay him.

I was put on the usual after-surgery liquid diet, which presented a problem. I was allergic to greasy broths, Jell-O, juices, tea, and coffee. When I asked for a pop or a cola, the nurse said no. It was a starvation diet.

Hospital noises, a feeling of numbness, concern over my recovery, all made me restless and made sleep difficult. The patient in the next bed had gallstone problems and kept calling for a shot for her pain. For some time, she got no response.

Finally, a nurse came into the room and said, "Here's your shot for pain, Mrs. Stevens."

"No! I don't get shots for pain! The lady in the next bed has been calling for pain medication." It had almost happened again!

"You'll have to excuse me," the nurse apologized. "We're on a twelve-hour shift. I'm tired and not thinking clearly right now."

Thank God I had been unable to sleep!

The next morning, the neurosurgeon, concerned that I had taken nothing by mouth, authorized the nurse to bring me anything I wanted. I asked for a plain salad with clear Italian dressing. It had to be fresh lettuce with nothing touching it, I told her. No tomatoes, cucumbers, radishes, or the like, I stated, telling her that I had severe allergic reactions to all those foods.

Thinking that my instructions had been followed, I ate the seemingly simple salad. Now, in addition to recovering from brain surgery, I also had diarrhea, stomach pains, and was going into shock, getting very cold. They obviously had taken an already assembled salad and removed the tomato, cucumbers and other vegetables, not believing how sensitive my allergies were.

"I want to go home where I will be safe," I told the neurosurgeon. It was only the day after surgery.

"No, you must stay in the hospital for several days."

"Either release me or I will sign myself out. I'm going home. I could be killed in here."

The next day, the doctor signed my release form and Bob took me home, where I would be safe in his care.

My forehead looked great and soon, I hoped, I would have no more pain. The good news was that this was not a return of a pituitary tumor, but other tumors and some damage apparently resulting from either the metal plate in my head or the extensive radiation that I had received over twenty years before.

Now, a new and unexpected problem arose. The insurance company informed me that the neurosurgeon had refused to sign the referral form needed to authorize payment to the plastic surgeon.

I went to the neurosurgeon's office. I was standing in the reception area, speaking to the doctor through the small window behind which the receptionist worked. I pushed the insurance form through the window and asked him to sign it.

"The insurance company needs your signature in order for Dr. Vasileff to be paid for the plastic surgery that he performed."

"I'm not signing that form. I didn't refer you to him."

"Either you sign that form or I will sue you for your incompetency in my surgery, when you failed to scrape the bone for tumor remnants."

He gave me a poisonous look, but reached through his window, took the form, signed it and shoved it back to me. I have never seen him since and, certainly, would never recommend him.

Life went on and in the fall of 1990, I was asked to chair the education committee for the local Board of Realtors. I had worked on that committee for years, so I agreed. Throughout the year of 1991, I MC'd many of the meetings. During this time, I always wore a scarf, which showed only a little bit of hair in the front and back of my head.

"Are you wearing a scarf in sympathy for the Arab war?" several of my colleagues asked me.

"No, I'm wearing it because I have a huge incision from ear to ear, and if you saw it, you would probably puke!" was my standard response.

I hated the pressure of a wig on my head, and the scarves provided an excellent solution. After the incision healed, my skin reacted to certain shampoos. My scalp blistered, not just at the incision, but all over my head. This reaction required me to select extremely mild shampoos, and even then, I had to dilute them. Since I couldn't use chemicals on my head, I could no longer bleach my hair to a white blond and perms were not possible. I let Mother Nature handle my hair coloring.

The year 1991 was also the year in which Bob and I returned to the altar and renewed our marriage vows. It was our twenty-fifth wedding anniversary.

"We got married for better or for worse, and all these years, I've only had the better. When do I get the worse?" Bob said to me during the ceremony.

Tears welled up in my eyes. Later, he told me that if he ever has heart surgery, they will find a note in his heart that says, "My heart belongs to Mary!" I do believe him.

Chapter 17

Blowing Bubbles

A side effect of the tumors in my forehead had been pressure on my eyes. Now, cataracts were developing. I always thought cataract surgery was for older people, but I was about to have the surgery on both eyes within a two year span.

I told the doctor, who performed the first surgery, about my allergies and that I needed to be given carbocaine, as an anesthetic. He said that he would take care of it on the day of the surgery. I gave him the names and phone numbers of both my allergist and my endocrinologist.

Obviously, he never called either of them. While I was being prepped for the operation, over my objections that I don't respond accurately to such tests, he did a skin test for marcaine. As my allergist would have told him, had he had the opportunity, the test indicated, incorrectly, that I was not allergic to the drug. He went ahead and used marcaine without my knowledge. Had I known, of course, I would have cancelled the surgery.

The anesthesiologist injected marcaine into my eye and tested to determine if the tissue was frozen. An inaccurate positive result told him that it was. The ophthalmologist began the surgery. I began to scream in pain. The eye tissue began to bleed into the eye, causing an emergency situation. They remedicated me and I slipped into unconsciousness.

In the middle of the night, I was rushed to a retina specialist, who said that if the bleeding had reached the back of the eye, I would have been in serious danger to the point of dying.

I recovered, but put the ophthalmologist on my list headed: "Don't go near this doctor again!"

109

Happily, the second surgery was performed without incident by an excellent doctor in Rochester Hills, who listened to me, believed me about my allergies and remained in constant contact with my allergist and endocrinologist. It's so easy when you have a doctor, who lacks arrogance, listens to the patient and really wants to help.

Remember the enlarged thyroid/goiter problem caused by my root disease, acromegaly? The goiter was growing internally into my throat area. One doctor didn't want to remove it, fearing it would cause me to lose my voice. I was then referred to a specialist at a university hospital, who only performed throat surgery. He wanted to remove the enlarged thyroid/goiter immediately, noting that the way the goiter was growing, they might later have to crack open my chest to get to it. As it was, in his words, he had to "pull it out of the chest area."

I didn't lose my voice, but after recovery, it did change, becoming even hollower sounding. On the positive side, I do have a voice; and, in addition to the good feeling of having the lump out of my throat, I could now lie flat in bed without a breathing problem.

Having the entire thyroid removed, meant that I will take medication for the rest of my life. It took some trial and error to arrive at the correct dosage of synthroid, but eventually, taking 0.15 milligrams for six days and then taking a day off, works fine. I feel great!

I wasn't out of the woods, yet. My allergies took a new twist. Dining in a steakhouse restaurant in South Bend, Indiana, I ordered a filet mignon, a steak that I usually could enjoy with no problems. I always attack the steak by cutting it through the middle, looking to be sure it is medium rare and checking for any signs of fat, which would cause me the old bug-a-boo of diarrhea, nausea and, sometimes, shock.

This steak looked gorgeous and very lean. I began to eat the steak in my usual manner, slicing small pieces from the middle and enjoying every bite. I enjoyed it, that is, until I sliced a piece out of the edge of the steak and put it in my mouth. Just touching it with my tongue, without even swallowing, caused a choking sensation. Instantly, without warning, my throat began to swell up and close over. I raced toward the bathroom holding my napkin over my mouth, choking and gasping for air.

Bob and my daughter came racing after me, got me to the car and rushed me to the emergency room of a nearby hospital. My voice sounded like Donald Duck's. I had difficulty breathing and couldn't swallow my saliva, which had become thick and bubbly. I continually spit it out for fear of drowning in it. As I did, I blew large bubbles. Anyone watching me would have thought I was chewing bubble gum!

"Is this your normal voice?" the emergency room doctor asked.

I shook my head, no. For about six hours, doctors and nurses shot various allergy drugs into me with an IV push after each one, until my heartbeat finally returned to normal, my blood pressure calmed down and the swelling in my throat subsided. By morning, I could once again swallow my saliva. The entire episode had been a totally new experience for me and extremely scary.

Apparently, what had happened was that the kitchen grills where the steaks and fish were prepared were side by side. The edge of my steak must have touched a piece of fish. As highly allergic as I am, that's all it takes.

From that day forward, Bob and I always ask at every restaurant, whether they grille or cook their steaks or chicken at the same location, as they do their fish. If they answer in the affirmative, I ask that they use foil or a separate pan for my steak. Most chefs have been cooperative.

A week later, dining at home, I placed a mushroom in my mouth. I love mushrooms and had never been allergic to them, but I was now. Touching my tongue to the mushroom caused the same reaction as I had to the piece of steak. Again, we raced to the hospital, while I experienced an identical throat seizure–pounding heart, gasping for breath, Donald duck voice, thick saliva, blowing bubbles. Again, it took hours for my body to calm down.

Terrifying me, a whole new list of foods began causing the same throat seizures–cauliflower, smoked meats, pork, corn, cheese and other milk products, almost all vegetables. The emergency room doctors advised Bob to call the paramedics, rather than drive me to the hospital.

My allergist had now semi-retired. Much as I would miss him, I found a new doctor, who prescribed three Epipens. An Epipen is an auto-injector of epinephrine; a drug used for allergic emergencies and is usually injected into the muscle of the thigh. He instructed me to give myself three injections, as soon as the seizure symptoms began. I did as he said, but while the injections made my body hyper, they did not reverse the allergic reactions.

Bob and I read the ingredients on all food packages before purchasing and cooking them. We have found that food processors change ingredients constantly, making it necessary to continually check the same item over and over.

Beside all the exterior physical changes that acromegaly or a pituitary disorder can cause, it can also damage internal organs– heart, liver, stomach or colon. Tests showed that my colon was enlarged, apparently a common occurrence in acromegaly patients. Because of my situation, I must be tested for the appearance of polyps in the colon area, which could become malignant. Colon cancer ran in my father's side of the family, which is a double reason for me to be tested.

When I have a colonoscopy performed, I present a double problem. Besides being allergic to the medications usually prescribed, my colon is enlarged–jam packed inside of my body– so doctors call me "curly." I am always anesthetized, as are most people today, so the additional pain I would otherwise sustain is not a problem.

In the spring of 1997, I began experiencing a bite change in my mouth. Are my top teeth and bone section moving inward causing pain around the upper portion of my teeth and nose, or is my jaw suddenly starting to jut out? My bottom teeth were extended farther out than my upper teeth, making it difficult to bite into foods. My internist/endocrinologist ordered a CAT scan without the dye to see if the pituitary tumor was returning.

The radiologist responded that there was a great deal of scar tissue, but no signs of a new tumor. I went into a "wait and see" mode. Within a year, my lower jaw and teeth commenced to move inward, causing pain, until the year 2000, when I finally had a natural bite. My dentist was amazed at the whole process. My husband, just remarked, "After brain surgery in 1968, I just wait, and over the years my wife keeps changing on me. I love it!"

While all this was happening in the late 90's I also began to feel pain in my knee joints. When I rolled over in my sleep and woke with knee pain, I knew it was finally time to see an orthopedic doctor. Acromegaly, I was told, can affect the cartilage between the bones, and that is what had happened. X-

rays showed that my knee joint was bone-on-bone with no cartilage between. As a result, in the year 2000, I had my right knee replaced and in the year 2001, the doctor replaced my left knee. Now, with a metal plate and metal clips in my head and metal knees, I should be called the "bionic woman." I wish I had her strength!

By spring of 2004, I experienced a bite change again. This time, the mouth change also affected the bridge work on my upper front teeth, and one tooth broke off at the gum line. My internist/ endocrinologist ordered another CAT scan with no dye to verify that the pituitary tumor was not returning. The radiologists responded in the negative, so I was just going through a bite change. I was shrinking.

My front bridge had been five teeth, now it would include six. The insurance company wanted a partial instead of a permanent bridge–it would be cheaper. Ever since the metal plate and metal clips were placed in my head in 1968, I had difficulty wearing metal earrings (they blistered my skin) and metal necklaces (they caused my neck to itch and sores to breakout). I wore necklaces only with turtleneck sweaters and that was great. A partial bridge was made and inserted into my mouth with the same results–blisters and sores in my mouth that would not heal.

I wrote a personal letter to the dental insurance company, stating my problems with metal and the need to change to a permanent bridge. The insurance company responded with, "Yes, they would pay their portion of the fee," which surprised the dentist, and now I have six teeth in a permanent bridge in my mouth. As I grow older, it seems that I am shrinking around the mouth. Will this happen again in the years to come? God only knows.

Chapter 18

Standing by Bob

"Mary, I don't feel too good," Bob said one day. "The right side of my face seems numb and my arm is numb."

With all the difficulties I was experiencing, my husband, my "Rock of Gibraltar," began to have problems, also. Although diabetic since 1980, Bob was usually in very good health. I was shaken when he walked into the kitchen on that day in November of 2004, and made this announcement; but I quickly stopped my dinner preparations and drove him to the emergency room at Beaumont Troy Hospital, just five miles away.

Test results showed that Bob was having mini strokes (TIA's) and had some blockage in the right carotid artery. The mini strokes stopped and the hospital doctor sent him home with a prescription for a blood thinner, after scheduling carotid artery surgery on the right side of the neck and head. We notified our family doctor, who insisted that Bob have a stress test first.

Thank God for the family doctor! The stress test revealed a blockage in his heart. The carotid artery surgery was canceled and a catheterization of his heart was ordered for the following Monday at the medical building adjoining Beaumont Hospital in Royal Oak. Bob and I were both grateful that this problem was discovered, and we definitely prayed for a good outcome.

During a heart catheterization, a doctor inserts a thin, plastic tube (catheter) into an artery or vein in the groin area and advances the tube into the chambers of the heart or the coronary arteries to check for blockage or other problems. Monday, Bob's catheterization had just begun and then it was over.

"We can't get into his heart for the catheterization." the doctor told, as I sat nervously in the waiting room. "His arteries are too blocked up. We are waiting for a room and he will be transported directly to the hospital and scheduled for open heart surgery."

Now, I really began to tremble. While waiting for the transfer, I called our children and Bob's cousins to alert them to the news and then I prayed and cried to my God. We really needed help!

As soon as we arrived in the hospital room, a cardiologist immediately joined us to discuss the surgery. Everything was moving so fast!

"You are scheduled for open heart surgery on Wednesday at 1:00 p.m." the doctor told Bob. "There is no guarantee that you will make it to Wednesday. You could take one step and drop dead."

He was trying to impress us with the seriousness of Bob's condition.

"When you get into my heart, you will find a note there that says, 'My heart belongs to Mary!'" Bob told him.

The doctor laughed. "I'll have to tell my wife that one!" he said.

When we were alone, Bob told me, "I won't take one step; I will take two!"

It wasn't funny. This was so serious. Just a week ago, Bob and I had made plans for a vacation to Branson. He appeared to be so well. We had no idea such a tremendous problem was hiding under the patina of good health.

The nurse came into the room and notified us of the barrage of tests scheduled for Tuesday. It was going to be a very busy day for Bob.

As I drove to the hospital on Wednesday morning, I began to pray out loud, shouting as loud as I could. "God, you know I need Bob! I love him and I need him! Please make this surgery successful. You have to help us, God we need your help!" People driving near me, must have wondered who I was shouting at, but I didn't care. I just wanted God to hear me and answer my prayers.

Our daughter, Gina, and Bob's cousins were there for my support. We could only wait and pray. A nurse came out periodically to notify us that the surgery was going well. Finally, the surgeon arrived.

"The surgery went fine," he told us. "We did five by-passes, two of them were clogged one-hundred percent and the other three at about ninety-five percent, plus he had a large hole in his heart. He is in recovery and since it is late in the day, the nurse will soon let you join him," he continued. "I don't know how that man was alive!"

I hugged the surgeon and said, "The power of prayer–God knows I need him. Thank you, doctor!"

As my relatives left, happy that everything had gone well, I was alone again with my God–saying, "Thank you, thank you," over and over again.

A short time later, I was admitted into the recovery room, where Bob was slowly coming out of the anesthetic.

When he could hear me, I told him, "Bob, you had a large hole in your heart!"

"I know how I got it." He looked at the nurse and then at me. "Cupid's arrow!"

Over the years, Bob had always been there for me–so reliable, so loving and caring. Now, it was my turn to be there for him, during his recovery.

In January, 2005, the carotid artery surgery was completed on the right side of his neck and head and my Bob was back to normal. No more blockages and hopefully, no more problems.

In the fall of 2005, we scheduled the Branson vacation as previously planned; however, Bob came down with contagious pneumonia and a partial lung collapse while in Branson, and we quickly returned home to Michigan for his recovery. Cold weather caused him to have chest pains, so next we planned a lengthy winter vacation in Fort Myers, Florida, where it was warm and so relaxing.

Upon returning to Michigan in March, the cold weather again caused Bob to have chest pains, probably from the partially collapsed lung. So in spring 2006, Bob and I made permanent plans to move to The Villages in Florida. We were amazed at how our plans fell into place. In the summer of 2006, we sold our house in Michigan, purchased a new house in The Villages, and by early September, we became permanent residents in Florida. We miss our relatives and friends in Michigan, but Bob's health is of prime importance.

Togetherness is so important. Together, Bob and I have taken golf lessons—so you will often find us in our golf cart heading to a nearby golf course or to a Village restaurant. We joined a nearby Catholic Church with many organizations that we can be a part of—ushering, teaching and assisting people in need. Of prime importance with this church is their constant format of worshiping God through the Mass and their many other opportunities for prayer and social life—important aspects for the people of God.

Are my food allergies getting worse? Yes, but we are accustomed to dealing with that. Excellent doctors—cardiologists, endocrinologists, pulmonary doctors, family doctors, dentists— Bob and I have had access to excellent doctors and this is also a blessing from God.

I'm pleased and grateful to have the best medical care for my "Rock of Gibraltar."

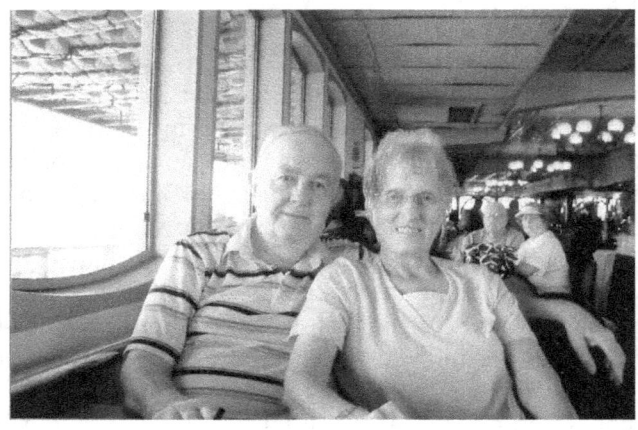

Bob and Mary Stevens

118

Chapter 19

A Blessing in Disguise

In the nineties, I began to think about my life with acromegaly, a pituitary disorder, and the severe allergy problems that I have experienced. I had read several articles on Rondo Hatton, a movie actor, who played roles as a monster and who had acromegaly. His facial disfigurement was so grotesque, he never needed makeup for his monster roles. Yet, when he had graduated from high school, he had been considered a handsome youth.

There are others diagnosed with acromegaly who have come to the attention of the press. Sandy Allen was one of these. At 7 feet, 7 inches tall, she was recognized as the world's tallest woman, until her death on August 13, 2008.

According to an Associated Press release, Allen's pituitary gland, which had been producing too much of the growth hormone, was operated on in 1977 in an effort to stop further growth.

In the eighties and nineties, I began to search for patients with acromegaly or pituitary disorders. My brain tumor was found by accident in the sixties, and my problem was definitely in my head. For me, the doctors indicated that I had no choice—surgery was my only option.

The purpose of this book is to bring public awareness of pituitary tumors and the damage that can result if never diagnosed. Acromegaly is a disease that can cause severe damage to a patient, even insanity and death. How many patients in insane asylums really have acromegaly?

Do not presume that a complete physical examination will discover a pituitary problem. It won't; you can trust me on this one. Most physical examinations do not include blood tests for levels of cortisol, prolactin and growth hormone. Often, the patient must request that these tests be performed.

I invite you to take a look at the Research section of the Appendix and read what several of these patients have to say.

Also, in the Appendix is a presentation for the layman of what to look for, if you think that you or a loved one might have a pituitary tumor. I am not a doctor and I don't pretend to speak here as one. These are my observations, arrived upon out of my own experience and frustration in my long search for a proper diagnosis.

In addition, I have prepared a glossary of some of the terms used throughout the book.

Finally, if reading this book had been of help to even one person with this puzzling disease, I will be grateful. I have been so blessed in my life; it would be my very great pleasure to help someone else in their quest.

Appendix

Mary J. Stevens

RESEARCH

Since my own involvement with acromegaly, I have become interested in the development of treatment for diseases of the pituitary gland. I know that neurosurgery has come a long way, with tremendous advances in various forms of radiation, use of the gamma ray knife, stereotactic fractionated radiosurgery, new medications, new health products, and new surgical techniques, but how about the patients?

How are people discovering whether or not they have pituitary tumors? What kinds of psychological problems affect these patients? Does their medication enhance their psychological problems or alleviate them? In my search for answers, I interviewed several patients with pituitary tumors. The experiences that I relate are real-life experiences which have come directly from those patients, not from their doctors. What they told me follows.

Beverley:

"It's a blessing in disguise."

These words spoken by a neurosurgeon, summarized the relief that Beverley and her husband felt just prior to her surgery for a pituitary tumor, she told me.

Other than her menstrual periods being erratic and beginning at a later age than most girls and continuing during her second pregnancy, Beverley told me that her other symptoms didn't begin until age 36, a year after a therapeutic abortion for a baby for whom there had been no heartbeat.

Her symptoms were: shortness of breath; weakness in her legs; general lethargy, accompanied by the feeling that energy was draining from her body; dry mouth and great thirst; extreme sensitivity to light, especially at night, when light appeared to her like lightning streaks; and hypoglycemia detected by a glucose tolerance test.

After she quit smoking, Beverley gained forty pounds and sought professional help. A neurologist performed an EEG (electroencephalogram), which showed that there were deteriorating cells of the sella, the bony structure that houses the pituitary gland. He recommended additional testing in a year's time. Beverley neglected to return for the tests.

Five years later, she again sought medical help, when her health problems worsened–constant exhaustion, difficulty breathing at night, a feeling as if her neck and head were swelling, a choking sensation when lying down, continued extreme sensitivity to light, and a ringing in the ears.

An ophthalmologist determined that her eye pressure was high (a forerunner of glaucoma), and her peripheral vision was off. He changed the prescription for her glasses and prescribed Betagan eye drops to combat the pressure problem.

After taking the medication for a year, her vision was worse; so Beverley returned to the neurologist, who ordered a blood test for white cell count (low) and a bone marrow (normal). He did not do a growth hormone study.

Beverley's complaints increased and her head seemed in turmoil. She responded by taking lots of aspirin. Since some of her complaints could now be attributed to menopause, they were ignored.

Some ten years later, Beverley noticed that her hands and feet were getting larger; then, she began coughing up blood clots. Her family physician gave her medication for diarrhea and vomiting and diagnosed her case as severe flu. How many times had that been my fate?

She had chills and felt terribly cold, talked nonsensically, was extremely thirsty, and had trouble seeing. The doctor told her husband that these symptoms were probably a reaction to the flu medication. He was reluctant to admit her to the hospital.

When Beverley passed out, her husband rushed her to a nearby hospital, where after several days of testing, A CAT scan showed the existence of a pituitary tumor. The neurosurgeon to whom she was referred, found that a cyst had apparently ruptured near the area of the pituitary tumor and caused her to cough up the blood clots. Had it not been for the cyst, her real problem, the pituitary tumor, would not have been discovered. It was a blessing in disguise; an accidental diagnosis, as I had experienced in my life.

After surgery, the fifty-five-year-old Beverley regained ninety-nine percent of her peripheral vision and her energy level increased. She refused the offer for radiation therapy to destroy any particles of the tumor that might remain. Because pituitary disorders can run in families, she has been advised to have her children tested.

Kimberly

"I diagnosed myself!"

Thirty-two-year-old Kimberly, a wife, mother and engineer grew nine-and-a-half inches in height within ten months at the age of twelve. The family doctor said that if the excessive growth didn't stop, she would require surgery on her pituitary gland. It did stop when she reached five-feet-seven-inches.

When she was thirteen, birth control pills were prescribed in an unsuccessful attempt to stabilize her erratic menstrual cycle. This seems to be one of the commonalities of a pituitary tumor.

At age seventeen, a milky discharge from her breast began and has continued until the present time. A year later, Kimberly married and a year after that, her first child was born. Drugs to relax the birthing muscles induced labor and allowed for a natural birth.

For the next few years, Kimberly experienced extremely irregular menstrual cycles, stopping for a couple of years and beginning again. During this time, she gave birth to two children, the first by induced labor and the last by a C-section, following hemorrhaging which put both mother and baby at risk.

One doctor diagnosed her problem as menopause and another said it was due to her emotions and nerves. "You cause your own problems," he said.

As I listened to Kimberly, I was thrown back to the days,

when these things were happening to me. But, unlike my inability to gain weight, Kimberly gained over fifty pounds, became pregnant again, and her fourth child was born after two days of induced labor.

In addition to her emotional problems, Kimberly was plagued with exhaustion; she noticed that her foot size changed from a size seven to a size nine and from narrow to wide. Her hands and fingers were enlarged with her ring size increasing two-and-a-half sizes. In addition, she had a larger over-bite, larger lips, and a protruding forehead. Severe headaches, loss of peripheral vision, extreme sweating, light sensitivity (especially at night), and a choking sensation when trying to sleep, were among her symptoms.

After doing research on her own, Kimberly suspected that she might have acromegaly. She presented the information to her doctor and he agreed with her, but tests bounced back and forth. It wasn't acromegaly; it was acromegaly. Finally, transphenoidal surgery for a pituitary tumor was performed at a reputable hospital.

Informed that all had gone well, Kimberly continued to have severe problems. Then came the bad news. The tumor had not been removed. What had been removed were some cysts.

For various reasons, an accurate diagnosis was not possible. Injections were prescribed, but after almost six months, her condition had not improved. Her shoe size continued to grow, extreme joint pain made walking difficult.

"Often I would have to crawl. Pain in (my) wrists made it a chore just to write my name," she said.

All the other symptoms, including weight gain and lactation continued.

"If I pressed on my breast, a stream of milk would shoot out from my body. It was so upsetting," Kimberly said

Ready to try anything, she began intensive research and heard of some intriguing health products.

She obtained literature and showed it to her doctor, who encouraged her to try them. She stopped the injections, which had seemed to be useless, and started taking the health products.

"Within a few weeks, I noticed a tremendous improvement. I had more energy and fewer painful headaches....the lactation in my breasts had completely stopped."

Tests soon reported excellent results.

"What are you taking?" her endocrinologist asked.

Kimberly responded, "Some health products."

Kimberly returned to work on a part-time basis. With this new-found natural product, Kimberly had a great deal of hope; however, it seemed her tumor had only been in remission and her pituitary problems did return.

Bill

Bill's behavior and appearance changed to such an extent that his marriage was at stake. He worked all week and spent weekends on the couch. He had gained weight and had no energy for family or household activities.

Shortly before the birth of their fourth child, his wife, Terri decided on a separation in order to maintain her own sanity and to protect the children. Bill's erratic emotional state had caused the family great stress, Terri told me, during the joint interview that I conducted with the couple.

As I sat listening to them outline Bill's symptoms, I felt as if I were hearing a record in my head. So many pituitary tumor patients' symptoms are similar, as are their doctor's reactions.

Bill's family doctor had told him that his overweight condition was his own fault.

"I won't take care of you, if you won't even take care of yourself," the doctor had said.

Bill had been checked for malaria, as a result of time spent in Thailand, and for HIV.

"I have been faithful to my wife one hundred percent," Bill said. It was humiliating for him to have been suspected as having HIV.

A gastroenterologist had identified marks on Bill's stomach as the striated marks of Cushing's disease, but his endocrinologist denied it.

A job performance report at work indicated that he was a workaholic and a report from his peer group stated that he was extremely aggressive and looked mean all the time.

"This made me realize," Bill said, "that Terri's fears relevant to my emotional state were probably quite valid. Obviously, I was a difficult person to get along with."

A group of doctors were scheduled to examine Bill to reach an opinion regarding his medical problems. He wanted Terri to attend the meeting to prove to her that he wasn't a hypochondriac; but, Terri thought it was a setup to try to coax her back into a relationship with Bill, and she refused to attend.

The doctors examined him, as he lay naked on the table.

"I felt like a piece of meat," Bill told me.

But the results were heartening. "You do have Cushing's disease," they reported and ordered an MRI which showed a pituitary tumor.

Then came the bad news. "You have only three to six months to live. We cannot contain your blood pressure," one doctor told him. "Either you will have a stroke or a catastrophic adrenal failure, since your body pumps out too much cortisol. You have the highest levels of cortisone that I have seen in twelve years. Besides the striated marks on your abdomen, you are beginning to grow a buffalo hump on your back, which is common to patients with Cushing's disease."

Transsphenoidal surgery performed by a neurosurgeon was successful.

While waiting for the surgery to take place, Terri said that she had prayed for a miracle.

"I just knew God was giving us direction. I worried and I prayed."

I could relate to that.

Even though Bill continued to have painful joints, his stamina had not returned and his vision was affected, both he and Terri see the surgery as a big success. Most of his symptoms disappeared, including the buffalo hump and the striated marks on the abdomen. The family is now happily reunited.

Bill learned of an organization, PNA (Pituitary Network Association), a support group that issues a Resource Book relating stories of patients with similar health problems. Bill told me that it has helped him to understand the vagaries of his disease.

Karen

During her teen years, Karen encountered severe headaches, allergies, sensitivity to light, a balance problem, continual thirst and she felt that her tongue was swollen in her mouth. In college, she added ongoing exhaustion. She was labeled as having chronic fatigue syndrome.

After meeting, falling in love with and marrying, fellow skier, Bill, she experienced three miscarriages and her symptoms increased, as others were added.

Eventually, doctors performed a partial colonectomy.

"They removed huge amounts of extra colon," Karen told me, "which they said could be precancerous. Then the doctors told me that my headache problems should be over. Not true."

Karen's story follows so many others: difficult pregnancies-her baby was premature, weighed only one and a half pounds and lived only eleven days; headaches; vision problems; allergies; abnormal growth in the face, hands and feet; and, finally, a diagnosis of acromegaly.

After surgery, Karen's problems continued with weight gain and stomach difficulties among others, and more surgery.

"It takes time to heal," doctors told her.

In 1993, I interviewed a vibrant, optimistic Karen, then thirty-nine years old. She said that so many problems still existed, but by her various comments, I knew that she had a great sense of humor and a strong fighting spirit. I was confident that she would improve. Karen related how fortunate she was to have Bill, a wonderful, loving and supportive husband.

I interviewed Bill and he updated me on Karen's surgeries. In 1995, he said he had realized that she needed his full-time care. He quit his position as an executive vice president of a large company, because a little voice told him that "Karen needs you at home."

Stomach surgery and complications hospitalized her from the fall of 1996 until spring of 1997. Now losing weight dramatically, doctors inserted a feeding tube, but her body rejected it.

On March 2, 1997, Karen died from multiple organ failures at forty-three years of age. There was standing room only at her funeral and seventy-seven cars in the procession, a fitting tribute to a woman who was never strong enough physically to hold down a job, but continually gave of herself to assist others, including working at the Michigan Cancer Foundation and the Rainbow Connection.

Gail

When she was two-years-old, Gail was tested for dwarfism. She had no neck; her head appeared to be sitting on her shoulders. Her physical problems began earlier than most acromegaly patients. By sixth grade, she was having vision problems, headaches and allergies.

After graduating from high school, Gail became a nurse's aid and married the love of her life, Terry, who ran the light show for a local band. When she was twenty, she was severely injured in a head-on collision. The driver of the other car was a boy, who had stolen his parents' car and was drunk. Gail died twice on the operating table, but survived, experiencing a slow recovery.

Her physical problems continued, but she was able to deliver a baby daughter normally. Afterward, because of menstrual difficulties and a dropped uterus, a hysterectomy was performed.

Told the usual, that she was stressed and nervous, Valium and then Premarin were prescribed.

Her hands were so enlarged, her rings had to be cut off of her fingers. Carpel tunnel preceded the enlargement, which was followed by weight gain and pain in various parts of her body
Other symptoms included dental problems, excessive jaw pain and an enlarged tongue. These difficulties became so severe, that it was necessary to place an occlusive guard on her top teeth to stop the pain and to stop her from grinding her teeth at night.

Gail's enlarged tongue collapsed while she slept and blocked her airway, causing her to struggle for breath, to sweat to the point of drenching the sheets, and finally to wake up. Her lack of sleep at night caused her to fall asleep on the job. Not a good thing for a nurse.

Doctors suggested cutting a "V" into her tongue, surgically reducing its size. She and Terry decided against this drastic action.

Heavy sweating became a problem.

"I worked as a scrub nurse in labor and delivery...I would feel the sweat under the cap, which would actually feel like it was sizzling on my scalp, that's how hot I felt," Gail told me.

Her physical condition continued to worsen with more and more new symptoms, until when she was forty-six years old, her family doctor discussed with her the possibility that she might have acromegaly. An MRI confirmed this diagnosis and surgery for the pituitary tumor was planned.

"I was an emotional wreck," Gail said, "trying to continue to work, knowing I had to face brain surgery."

After the operation, Terry asked if the surgeon had removed the entire tumor.

"I didn't remove the entire tumor," he said, "because I didn't want to nick the carotid artery and couldn't go as far up as I wanted to because I couldn't see it. The spot of tumor that was left was about the size of a dime."

Radiation therapy reduced the size of the remnants of the tumor. Gail's skin tissue, nose, tongue, lips, hands and feet all decreased in size. She knows she still has a brain tumor but is relieved that her appearance has become more normal.

A new symptom that she must face is memory loss, making it difficult to return to classes in pursuit of her nursing degree. Another troublesome detail is that after surgery, her endocrinologist appeared to be too busy to listen to her needs.

Unfortunately, this is not uncommon and when it occurs, the best thing to do is what Gail did: Find a new doctor. This is not as easy as it sounds. The patient is tired and in pain and doesn't need one more chore to add to the list, but it's a better solution that staying with an unfeeling physician. This is also the reason why a caring advocate, such as Gail's husband, Terry, is so important.

Gail, still a tiny person at four feet ten inches tall, continues to have physical difficulties and recommends support groups for anyone in her position.

"We would recommend to anybody with pituitary problems to join a support group. You can gain so much knowledge through interaction with other pituitary patients, as well as from the various presentations by numerous medical doctors and nurses," was Gail's final comment to me.

Lori

Even in childhood, weight was a problem for Lori, whose menstrual cycle began at age twelve and was always irregular. After college, she entered the world of work, but knew something was wrong by her heavy fatigue and susceptibility to colds and sinus infections.

"When driving home from work, which was only about twenty miles, I had to open the window of the car in order to get fresh air to help stay awake," Lori told me. "When that didn't work, I would take off my shoes, so that the unique feeling of the pedal on my bare foot might irritate me enough, so I would stay awake while driving."

Sometimes, when she walked into the house, she would lie down and fall asleep still wearing her winter coat.

Three doctors dispensed similar advice: "Don't eat sugar; don't drink coffee; exercise; and try to lose weight."

This advice was for a woman who needed five alarm clocks to wake her up in the morning and, because even that sometimes didn't do it, she asked her mother, who lived across the state, to call her every day to make sure she was up!

Finally, a CAT scan revealed a pituitary tumor and she was put on experimental drug to reduce or eliminate it. The medication made her nauseated increased her weight and for about three months, her hair fell out. After two years of the drug and barely tolerating its side effects, an MRI indicated that the tumor had disappeared. Excellent! Except that the tumor returned–two more times.

"I have been very proactive this time around with my third tumor," Lori told me. "I did a survey on the Internet of one hundred people with pituitary tumors. I began the project when I was at my all time low, and it actually helped to pull me around and land me back on my feet."

She had thought that she was the only one who could understand the problems that she experienced or who could relate to the fear and feelings that she had carried around for eight years. Now, after communicating with all those people with pituitary tumors, she realized that many people shared a common experience with her.

"I keep in touch with so many pituitary patients now, and daily, I receive letters of support, letters of fear, and some that are pure inquiry. It keeps me busy responding to the email and supplying information to those who request it."

Lori learned how to build a web site for the sole purpose of reaching out to others.

"My web site had been well received," she said, "and is linked to the Brain Tumor Ring of Hope in England. Several thousand people have visited my site...My favorite part...is the page that lists individuals with pituitary disorders. There is a brief background about each person and an email address, so others can contact them. Nothing can replace the human touch in handling this problem." (At the time of the publication of this book, Lori's web site address was: http//members.aol.com/ tomajestic.)

At the end of our interview, Lori said, "It has taken me eight years to finally realize that it may be a blessing that I have prolactinoma, because I have learned so much about my self, and found that deep inside me, there is a strong girl that can 'hang with the best of them in the face of a challenge.' I learned a great deal about my ability to communicate with others, and extend the hand of friendship. For years, I kept everything bottled up inside of me, and now, it is great to be able to stand tall and be proud of myself, which I am."

Theresa

Although her tumor was not found until Theresa was in her mid-thirties, she had begun to experience its effects as young as sixteen. This is a fairly typical pattern for a patient with a pituitary disease.

"I had a really poor immune system–lots of viruses, mononucleosis and meningitis. By the time I turned twenty, I had a long medical history and a lot of unanswered questions."

In 1995, an MRI revealed a half-inch tumor on her pituitary gland. In spite of this and other symptoms, "No immediate medical intervention was taken," she reports.

After a year of physical and mental stress for Theresa and her family, partly due to her being made to feel like a hypochondriac, and partly due to the fight she put up to convince her doctors to order more tests, a comprehensive endocrine test led to the additional diagnosis that Teresa had Cushing's disease, a symptom caused by prolonged exposure and over-activity of the ACTH (corticotropic hormone that regulates the adrenal glands) secreting from the pituitary tumor.

In addition to the physical pain and weakness, the disease caused Teresa's dress size to increase from a size five to a twelve.

"By the fall of 1996," she says, "I was too ill to care for my family or even answer the phone without gasping for breath."

Finally, months later, with the pituitary tumor dangerously close to her optic nerve, causing a threat to her eyesight, Teresa underwent surgery.

Life after the diagnosis and surgery: She no longer has Cushing's disease and is now a size four. The dosage of the hormone replacement drug the doctor prescribed is down and, at the time of this interview, she anticipated that it would be lowered even further in the future. The down side is that she still experiences headaches, fatigue and neck and joint pain. She expected to resume a higher quality of life than has happened.

Although her recovery has been slow, she has embarked on a new journey. Theresa now reaches out to the community to educate people about pituitary tumors and their related diseases through a support group at a local hospital.

ACROMEGALY

My experience with acromegaly indicates that it is usually caused by a benign pituitary tumor. The word acromegaly comes from the Greek words for extremities and enlargement. From my experience and in my research, I have found that term reflects the most common symptom, the abnormal growth of the hands and feet. The patient frequently notices shoe size changes or rings that do not fit any more. If the growth begins as a child, it usually results in the child becoming a giant or a dwarf. Life expectancy for a giant seems to be very low. If the tumor is activated during puberty or in adult life, it can cause many serious complications and even reduce life expectancy.

The pituitary gland is a small bean-shaped gland located at the bottom of the brain and behind the eyes in the center of the head. It is connected by a stalk that is suspended from the hypothalmus. Together these two regulate how much of various hormones are produced according to your body's needs, which vary according to the time of day. The pituitary gland is often called "the master gland."

Pituitary tumors are often linked to kidney failure, cardiovascular problems, reproductive problems (infertility) in both men and women, cessation of the menses, vision impairment, eating disorders, and mood and behavioral disorders. A pituitary tumor does not cause all of these problems. The results will vary, according to the direction of the growth of the tumor.

Often misdiagnosed as a part of menopause or considered to be caused by a state of depression, hysteria, or a weight problem, a pituitary disorder is often completely ignored. If several of the problems listed above seem evident, contact your family doctor, an endocrinologist, or a neurologist to determine if the condition exists. I don't suggest that you become a hypochondriac, but real problems should not be ignored.

Blood tests, growth studies, and/or MRI or CAT scans can quickly determine if a pituitary disorder is present. Today, the condition can be treated by a variety of approaches, including oral medication to reduce the tumor, by gamma knife radio-surgery, by fractionated stereotactic radiosurgery, radiation therapy or by transphenoidal surgery. Although rare, a large tumor can be treated by a craniotomy type of surgery. As research continues, newer and more exciting innovations will be discovered.

Acromegaly is most frequently diagnosed during middle age. It occurs in both men and women.

Symptoms of Acromegaly

According to the Pituitary Tumor National Association's Resource Book, acromegaly is a chronic, insidious, debilitating disease resulting in serious cosmetic changes and metabolic complications. Apart from the coursening of facial features, the metabolic abnormalities associated with GH (Growth Hormone) hypersecretion are mainly responsible for increased cardiovascular mortality and warrant effective GH lowering therapy.

Physical Changes

Before puberty, the person may show dwarfism or excessive growth or extreme height known at giantism; however, after puberty the person may still experience inappropriate growth, which can be of the fingers, hands, feet, jaw, eye ridges, or head. Soft tissue growth can be either external, such as enlargement of the pads of the fingers or swelling of the feet, or internal with virtually every internal organ being enlarged.

Growth of the jaw may lead to separations or big gaps between the teeth. The tongue may grow and become very wide and more furrowed. Sometimes the tongue will begin to swell when the mouth is open. This should be noticed by your dentist.

Complications among those having the disease for any length of time arise from various cardiovascular problems, such as enlarged heart and attending blood supply system, or colon cancer. These two are the leading causes of death among acromegalics.

Symptoms of an Acromegaly Tumor

According to the PTNA Resource Book, the symptoms of an acromegaly tumor are:

* Oily skin; skin discoloration or darkening; skin odor due to excessive sweating
* Coarse facial features; enlargement of the lower lip, and of the tongue that eventually can lead to slurred speech; thickening and toughening of the skin; enlargement of the nasal passages; thickened ribs creating a barrel chest
* Vision impairment and/or blindness; vision defects; often limited peripheral vision; extreme sensitivity to lights, especially at night
* Dry mouth and heavy urination, often resulting in diabetes or hypoglycemia; enlarged saliva glands
* Deeper, hollower sounding voice due to enlargement of the vocal chords, often a choking sensation because of enlargement of vocal chords or thyroid
* Sleep apnea; drooling when asleep or awake
* Thyroid gland swelling and/or other thyroid problems, including signs of a goiter
* Eye ridges thicken, and eyes look deep set with prominent brow, called frontal bossing
* Hirsutism, or excessive hair growth on arms, legs, shoulders, face, chest, and back
* Loss (weakening) of cognitive abilities and/or memory lapses, may lead to insanity
* Low vitality (fatigue); unusual tiredness or loss of energy
* Headaches, from mild to severe, even migraine
* Carpel tunnel syndrome, with numbness, weakness or

tingling sensation in the hands
* Osteoarthritis or pain in the joints
* Loss of sexual interest (libido)
* Enlarging of hands (ring size), feet (shoe size), head (hat size), jaw (larger overbite or overbite); spreading of teeth
* Interrupted menstrual cycle; impotence
* Depression, irritability, anxiety attacks (psychological problems), mood swings, inability to control emotions, hypertension, apathy, short-term memory loss, personality changes, nervousness, and dizziness

Symptoms of a Prolactinoma Tumor
(prolactin = milk hormone)

A Prolactinoma, according to the PTNA Resource Book, is a tumor on the pituitary gland that secretes the milk hormone. The tumor is usually benign (noncancerous) ninety-nine percent of the time. It is the most common of all pituitary tumors (twenty-eight percent). The cause of the tumor is unknown.

Symptoms:

* Changes in menstrual cycle or loss of cycle (amenorrhea)
* Milk discharge (galactorrhea)
* Reduction in sex drive
* Pain on intercourse/vaginal dryness
* Headaches
* Visual field disturbances
* Male hypogonadism/impotence (shrinking testicles), milk discharge and enlargement of breast tissue in men
* Extreme mood changes and depression

Cushing's Disease

The PTNA Resource Book reports that Cushing's disease is caused by prolonged exposure of the body's tissues to high levels of the hormone cortisol. Cortisol is normally produced by the adrenal glands, which are just above the kidneys. Deficiency in cortisol can lead to low blood pressure, headache, nausea, vomiting, and even death.

Scientists think that normal cortisol levels help to:

* maintain blood pressure and cardiovascular function,
* slow the immune system's inflammatory response,
* balance the effects of insulin in breaking down sugar,
* regulate the metabolism of proteins, carbohydrates and fats
* and help the body respond to stress

Symptoms of Cushing's Disease

* Rapid, unexplained weight gain with rounding of the face (moon face and large, distended stomach, but usually thin extremities
* Buffalo hump (a collection of fat between the shoulders) and increased fat in the neck
* Skin changes–cheeks often red; acne or superficial skin infections; easy bruising
* Excessive hair growth on females
* Purple or bluish red striated marks on thighs, abdomen, buttocks, breasts, arms, and armpits similar to stretch marks
* Menstrual disorders in women; impotence in men
* Decreased fertility or absent libido (sex drive) in men
* High blood pressure, diabetes, and elevated temperature
* Excessive fatigue; decreased muscle strength
* Severe depression and/or psychosis
* Mood behavior disorders

Glossary

Acromegalic: Giantism.

Acromegaly: A hormonal disorder usually resulting from a benign pituitary tumor where the pituitary gland produces. an excess of a growth hormone (GH).

Adenoma: A benign tumor of a glandular structure.

Adrenal Gland: A pair of endocrine glands that produce small quantities of sex hormone.

Anesthetic: A substance that produces a general or local insensitivity to pain and other sensations, induced by a drug, such as ether, chloroform, gas, etc.

Anesthesiologist: A physician trained in administering anesthetics (drugs used during surgery or tests to prevent pain either by numbing a small area or causing unconsciousness).

Amenorrhea: Failure of a woman to menstruate.

Angiogram: A diagnostic test done in the x-ray department to visualize blood vessels after a contrast material has been introduced into the artery.

Benign: Noncancerous.

Biopsy: Removal and examination of a small amount of tissue taken from the body of the patient to make a diagnosis.

Bromocriptine: Inhibits prolactin secretion (Parlodol).

Cancer: Malignant tissue that destroys healthy tissue and tends to spread to other locations in the body.

Carcinoma: A malignant tumor found in the body tissue or organs. Tends to spread (metastasize) to other organs.

Catheter: A flexible, tubular surgical instrument inserted into body cavities or blood vessels for the insertion or removal of fluids.

CAT scan: Computerized axial tomography: An x-ray machine linked to a computer that produces an image of a certain cross-section of the body. A special dye is usually injected into the patient's vein prior to the scan to help to clarify the image.

Cauterize: Use of heat to seal wounded blood vessels and prevent uncontrolled bleeding.

Cavernous sinuses: Two irregularly shaped venous sinuses on each side of the sphenoid bone in the middle cranial bones which is a dilated channel for the passage of blood.

Cerebral: Referring to the cerebrum.

Cerebrosppinal fluid: The clear fluid made in the ventricular cavities of the brain that bathe the brain and the spinal cord. It circulates the ventricles and the subrachnoid space.

Cerebrum: The largest area of the brain that occupies the upper most part of the skull. It consists of two halves called hemispheres. Each half of the cerebrum is further divided into four lobes: frontal, temporal, parietal and occipital.

Chemotherapy: The use of chemical agents to treat tumors.

Cortisone: A steroid hormone secreted by the cortex (outer layer) of the adrenal gland, which is located on the kidneys.

Craniectomy: Surgery performed on the skull when pieces of bone are removed to gain entry to the brain and are not replaced.

Craniotomy: Surgery on the skull where a portion of bone is removed to gain access to the brain and the bone; metal or plastic is put back in its place.

Corticotropin (ACHT): Hormone that stimulates cortisol secretion (adrenal glands).

Cushing's disease: Hormonal disorder caused by prolonged levels of cortisol (e.g., excessive use of Prednisone); overproduction of cortisol by the body or more commonly by a pituitary tumor.

141

Cyst: A fluid filled mass or sac (often enclosed by a membrane).

Dexamethasone: A glucocorticosteroid medication used to reduce brain tissue swelling.

Diabetes insipidus: A problem with water balance in the body causing excessive urine production and great thirst, due to pituitary or hypothalamic damage.

Diabetes mellitus: Same symptoms as above due to not enough insulin production by the pancreas.

Diplopia: Double vision.

Dopamine agonists: Medications with predominant effects on pituitary cells that harbor receptors for the chemical transmitter dopamine.

Electroencephalogram (EEG): A graphic picture of the electrical activity of the brain made by placing electrodes (small terminals which conduct an electric current) on the person's scalp connecting the electrode wires to a machine called an electroencephalograph, which receives the pattern of the brain wave.

Encephalitis: Inflamation of the brain tissues (as a disease, it is most well known as sleeping sickness).

Endocrine glands: Those parts of the body that produce and secrete (release) hormones.

Endocrinology: The scientific study of dealing with the hormonal secretions of the glands, especially relating to their process and function.

Endometriosis: The presence of uterine lining in other pelvic organs, especially the ovaries, charactericized by cyst formation, adhesions and menstrual cramps.

Follicle stimulating hormone (FSH): A gonadotrophin hormone secreted by the pituitary gland, which promotes fertility (sperm production) in men and helps to regulate the menstrual cycle (follicle development) in women.

Gamma knife: A revolutionary noninvasive brain surgery procedure, also called radiosurgery, which allows surgeons to operate on abnormal areas of the brain with radiation using highly sophisticated computer technology to destroy targeted lesions while sparing surrounding tissue.

Gland: an organ of the body that produces materials (hormones) released into the blood stream, such as the pituitary or pineal gland. Hormones influence metabolism and other body functions.

Glucocorticosteroids: Medications used to decrease swelling around tumors. Medication to duplicate the effects of cortisol.

Goiter: An enlargement of the thyroid gland on the front and sides of the neck.

Gonad: A gland which produces the male and female reproduction cells—the testes (the spermatozoa) or the female ovaries (the ova).

Gonadotrophin: A hormone which regulates the function of the gonads; the two main gonadotrophins are LH and FSH, both released from the pituitary gland.

Gonadotrophin—releasing hormone (GnRH): Secreted by the hypothalamus, GnRH stimulates the release of LH and FSH from the pituitary gland.

Growth hormone (GH): A hormone produced by the anterior part of the pituitary gland that causes body growth.

Hirtsutism: Excessive hairiness in various parts of the body (most noticeable on the face).

Hormones: Chemical messengers that regulate bodily processes such as growth, reproduction, metabolism, digestion, mineral and fluid balance and the functioning of various organs.

Hyperlipidemia: Presence of excessive fats or lipids in the blood.

Hypoglycemic: An abnormally low level of glucose in the blood.

Hypogonadism: The inability of the gonads to function normally.

Hypopituitarism: Diminished activity of the pituitary gland, especially of the anterior lobe.

Hypothalamus: Located by the pituitary gland, controls such activities as body temperature, sexual drive,

appetite, blood glucose levels, moods and sleep/

arousal behavior patterns; it links the neural and endocrine systems to the pituitary gland, where the neural and hormonal systems interact.

Hypothyroidism: The condition produced by a deficiency of thyroid secretion, resulting in goiter, myxedema, and in children, cretinism.

Insulinlike growth factor (IGF-1): Produced in the liver.

Larynx: A muscular, cartilaginous structure lined with mucous membrane at the upper part of the trachea in which the vocal cords are located.

Larynx: A muscular, cartilaginous structure lined with mucous membrane at the upper part of the trachea in which the vocal cords are located.

Laser: An acronym of light amplification by stimulated emission of radiation. A surgical tool that creates intense heat and power when focused at close range, destroying cells by vaporizing them.

Lethargy: Sluggishness, drowsiness, fatigue.

Luteinizing hormone (LH): Secreted by the pituitary gland, promotes masculinity (testosterone production) in men and helps to regulate the menstrual cycle (ovulation) in women in conjunction with FSH.

Magnetic resonance imaging (MRI): A scanning device that uses a magnetic field, radio waves and a computer. Signals emitted by normal and diseased tissue during the scan are assembled into the image.

Novocain: A local anesthetic (painkiller) used by doctors.

Octreotide acetate: A steroid drug (sandostatin), used to reduce brain tumors.

Osteoporosis: A condition characterized by weakened and brittle bones, arising from a hormonal imbalance (also known as brittle bone disease).

Parlodol: A bromocriptine mesylate, taken orally is used to treat Parkinson's disease and to modulate the secreting a prolactin inhibitory factor (thought to be dopamine) to reduce or prevent breast milk production.

Pituitary gland: A small oval endocrine gland attached to the brain and located behind the eyes. This gland is the central controller in the regulation of secretions from many other hormone-secreting glands of the body. Half of the gland comes down from the brain (the posterior lobe, which controls the body's water levels and secretes the hormone ADH—anti-diuretic hormone). The other portion, the anterior lobe, controls sex hormone levels, growth hormone, lactation, body steroids and the thyroid gland.

Pituitary stalk: A tiny structure connecting the hypothalamus to the pituitary gland.

Progesterone: A sex hormone that is made in the ovaries and during pregnancy by the placenta.

Prolactin: Hormone released by the pituitary gland that activates the production of milk.

Prolactinoma: A tumor on the pituitary gland that secretes the milk hormone.

Radiation therapy: The use of radiation energy to interfere with the growth of a tumor.

Radiosurgery (stereotactic radiosurgery): A radiation therapy technique that uses a large number of narrow, precisely aimed, highly focused beams of ionizing radiation. The beams are aimed from many directions circling the head and meeting at a specific point.

Sandostatin (octreotide acetate): Taken by injection to reduce the size of a pituitary tumor.

Stalk: A stem. Usually refers to the pituitary stalk that connects the pituitary gland to the hypothalamus.

Steroids: See glucocorticosteroids.

Striated: Marks with a narrow furrow, ridge, stripe or streak.

Testosterone: The main male sex hormone, its production encouraged by LH from the pituitary gland. Small amounts are also present in women.

Thyroidectomy: Removal of all or part of the thyroid gland located in the throat.

Thyroid gland: An endocrine gland located on each side of the trachea connected below the larynx by a thin isthmus of tissue, the secretion of which regulates the rate of metabolism and growth.

Thyroid stimulating hormone (TSH): Regulates the function of the thyroid gland.

Trachea: The tube (windpipe) in people and all air-breathing animals extending from the larynx to the bronchi and is the principal passage for conveying air to and from the lungs.

Transsphenoidal: Surgery performed through the nostrils or a section of the mouth, usually extending through the sphenoidal sinus cavity into the pituitary area.

Tumor: An abnormal growth—may be benign or cancerous.

Ultrasound: Visualization of structures in the body by recording the reflections of sound waves directed into tissues. May be used during surgery.

Vascular: Relating to blood vessels.

Zoloft: Taken orally; often used to treat depression or obsessive-compulsive disorder.

* Note: Some articles (complete or in part) have been taken from *The Pituitary Patient Resource Guide* Second Edition, published by the Pituitary Network Association (PNA).

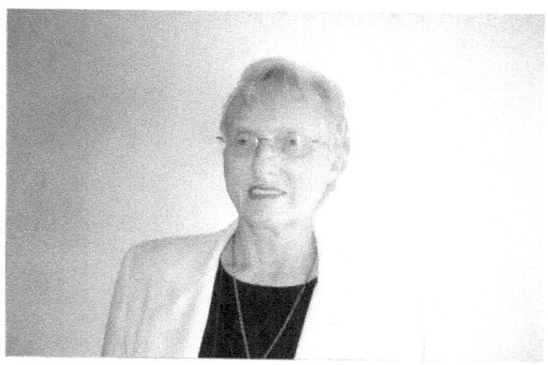

Mary J. Stevens who, while still dealing with aspects of acromegaly, especially a variety of allergies, now lives a busy and rewarding life in The Villages, Florida with her husband, Bob.

Mary believes that her life experiences, including recovery from brain surgeries and an "out of body" experience were all fantastic blessings from God, Who is intertwined in her life.

After describing the gradual physical distortions that she experienced, changing her forever from her identical twin, Mary has left all that behind her and lives in the present enjoying every moment of life that she shares with Bob. Today, she is a Christian, involved with her church in worshiping God, teaching catechism and assisting people in need.

She enjoys golfing, bowling and attending music festivities in the center of The Villages, not to mention dining at many exciting restaurants in the area that will cater to her needs. She looks forward to each day of her life with all the joys and surprises that await her—just knowing that God is at her side.

The purpose of the book is in Mary's words "not only to educate people on pituitary tumors but also to stress that no matter what problems you must face—physical, mental social, economic—stay positive in your attitudes and actions, and let God be a part of your life."

www.ingramcontent.com/pod-product-compliance
Lightning Source LLC
Chambersburg PA
CBHW070141290526
45789CB00002B/573